Healing Tuberculosis in the Woods

Healing Tuberculosis in the Woods

Medicine and Science at the End of the Nineteenth Century

David L. Ellison

Contributions in Medical Studies, Number 41

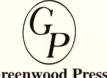

Greenwood Press
Westport, Connecticut • London

Library of Congress Cataloging-in-Publication Data

Ellison, David L.
    Healing tuberculosis in the woods : medicine and science at the
end of the nineteenth century / David L. Ellison.
        p.   cm.—(Contributions in medical studies, ISSN 0886–8220 ;
    no. 41)
    Includes bibliographical references and index.
    ISBN 0–313–29005–9 (alk. paper)
    1. Tuberculosis—History—19th century   2. Trudeau, Edward
Livingston, 1848–1915. I. Title. II. Series.
    RC310.E45   1994
    616.9′95′009034—dc20
    [B]   94–13689

British Library Cataloguing in Publication Data is available.

Library of Congress Catalog Card Number: 94–13689
ISBN: 0–313–29005–9
ISSN: 0886–8220

First published in 1994

Greenwood Press, 88 Post Road West, Westport, CT 06881
An imprint of Greenwood Publishing Group, Inc.

Printed in the United States of America

The paper used in this book complies with the
Permanent Paper Standard issued by the National
Information Standards Organization (Z39.48–1984).

10 9 8 7 6 5 4 3 2 1

Copyright Acknowledgment

The author gratefully acknowledges permission to quote from the following copyrighted
material:

Michael E. Teller, *The Tuberculosis Movement*. Reprinted with permission of Greenwood
Publishing Group, Inc., Westport, CT. Copyright © 1988.

Contents

Acknowledgments

The idea for this book came from a variety of places in my background.

My mother, Ione Benson Ellison, grew up in Saranac Lake in the sanitarium era. As a result I gulped my daily tablespoon full of cod-liver oil, slept with the window wide open in a dust-free home, never spit in her presence, and tested positive for tuberculosis, but never experienced the disease. Whenever I was sick for any reason, rest and good food were considered the most appropriate remedies.

My curiosity about Edward Trudeau as a person came from reading his autobiography and my general interest in tuberculosis. When I realized that his lifetime coincided with one of the major paradigm shifts in modern medicine, my general interest in the sociology of science began to take over. For that interest I am indebted to my teachers, Walter Hirsch and Robert Eichhorn, and my colleagues in the Science and Technology Studies Department at Rensselaer Polytechnic Institute.

All my life I have visited the Adirondack woods and the Saranac Lakes, enjoyed their beauty and felt restored after a stay of any length. Currently, I vacation one lake away (by boat) from the village. This made the research for this book particularly pleasurable. For the last few summers I have had the privilege of living at camp, driving my boat to Crescent Bay, and riding my bicycle to the Trudeau Institute or the Saranac Lake Free Library.

At the Institute I have benefitted from the extensive archives and records of the Sanitarium and the Saranac Laboratory. For this opportunity I would like to thank the Trudeau Institute and Mrs. Helen Jarvis, Librarian.

The Saranac Lake Free Library houses a fine collection of Adirondack Mountain records in its Adirondack Room. I appreciate the always friendly and knowledgable help of Mrs. Janet Decker and her able group of volunteers.

Historic Saranac Lake provided me with answers to many questions. Mary B. Hotaling allowed me to read one of her papers on Trudeau and made helpful suggestions on a part of the manuscript.

Local libraries at Albany Medical College and the New York State Health Department have been the sources of medical journals published in the nineteenth century.

The Rensselaer Polytechnic Institute Library has been extremely helpful, and I am especially appreciative of the help of Mrs. Jean Houghtaling at the interlibrary loan department.

I am very fortunate to work in a cordial and supportive academic department. For this I am grateful to our chair, Professor Shirley Gorenstein. Two assistants, Kathleen Ward and Linda Langford, were very helpful with the library research. At various times I have appreciated the secretarial support of Cathy Burniche, Linda Jorgensen, Carol Halder, Margaret McLeod, Kathy Vumbacco, and Christine Wigton.

When one lives with someone it is a major understatement to adequately account for or appreciate her contributions. Carolyn L. Olsen, Ph.D., my spouse, has read parts of the manuscript and encouraged my effort in countless ways. Without the happiness provided by our relationship, this book would not have been so much fun.

I would also like to thank Dr. James Sabin of Greenwood Press and the Production Editor, Terri M. Jennings, for many helpful suggestions. The final product, of course, is my responsibility.

Healing Tuberculosis in the Woods

1

Introduction

Thursday, November 18, 1915, in the small village of Saranac Lake, New York, and at Paul Smith's, another hamlet fourteen miles away, all operations were suspended, manufacturing stopped, and business houses closed their doors by decree of the Village Board. After his death Monday morning, November 15, the Village Board had appointed a committee to prepare a "resolution of respect embodying the regret of the Board at the death of Dr. Edward L. Trudeau, Saranac Lake's first village president and most prominent citizen" (*Adirondack Enterprise*, November 17, 1915). It was recommended that all flags be flown at half-mast until the burial. The greatness of the man was impressed upon the minds of the children by the closing of the schools for a half day. *The Adirondack Enterprise* announced that it was suspending the usual custom of charging to print resolutions of respect and would print all resolutions "prepared by any and every society upon the life and works of Dr. Edward L. Trudeau without charge."

The community of about 5,000 people recognized the worldwide importance of this man. He was described as "the beloved physician" by Stephen Chalmers (1916), a reporter from *The New York Times* who was sent to Saranac Lake to regain his health in 1908. In the previous thirty years Trudeau had made the village famous for the treatment of tuberculosis, a disease that killed one in seven Americans in the 1880s. Ironically they were honoring a man who attracted thousands of contagious invalids into their community. From the perspective of 100 years this seems preposterous. Would a physician be honored today for attracting AIDS patients with a less contagious disease to his community in hopes of sound medical advice and a possible cure?

Dr. Trudeau's death brought recognition from outside this small area of lakes in New York State's Adirondack Mountains. John Shaw Hoey wrote in the *Saranac Lake News* (November 15, 1915): "From the lowliest factory hut to the palatial mansion of the wife of a former Ambassador to the Court of St. James [a former patient, Mrs. Anson Phelps Stokes], from the poorest fireside to the richest home in the land will rise a silent prayer for the mercy of the soul of this great man."

A resolution was introduced before the Episcopal Diocese of Albany by Reverend Scott Kidder, Rector of St. Luke's, and seconded by Walter H. Cluett, lay delegate. Mr. Cluett had given up the presidency of his father's famous shirt factory in Troy, New York, to live with his tuberculous wife in Saranac Lake, where he eventually entered the real estate business.

Whereas the passing of Edward Livingston Trudeau, Doctor of Medicine, Doctor of Laws, Warden of the Mission of St. John's in the Wilderness, Paul Smith's and Senior Warden of the Church of St. Luke the Beloved Physician, Saranac Lake in the Diocese of Albany leaves a vacancy not only in the roll of this convention, but also in that of world wide known healers of the sick, be it Resolved that the Diocese of Albany give expression to its sense of such loss, to its appreciation of his unique and heroic life of service, and to its sympathy for his bereaved family and co-workers, by a silent and a rising vote (Scrapbook 10, p. 6).

The *Troy Times* said, "His method of treating incipient consumption has come to be widely recognized as the most reliable and successful, and campaigns against the 'white plague' now are waged largely along the lines which he originally marked out" (Scrapbook 10, p. 15).

New York City papers praised Trudeau also. *The New York Times* said

In the history of medicine . . . there must be recorded the names of not a few men to whose achievements will be accorded, and deservedly, more space than can be given there to those of Edward Livingston Trudeau. But none will get, or will have earned, sincerer recognition for elevation of character or for the dauntless courage and tireless energy, with which for forty years, he sought not in vain, to save others from the death that for all that time, as he well knew, might have come to himself on any day. . . .

There are senses in which he was not a great doctor, but none in which he was not a great man. Thousands owe their life to him, and millions more will do so. That they will not know it makes little difference, nor would it have troubled him at all, for a more modest, undemanding, simple living hero never walked the earth (Scrapbook 10, p. 15).

These sentiments were echoed by the *New York Globe*, the *Evening Post*, and the *Evening Sun*. A *Boston Herald* editorial noted that 500 sanitoria in this country and Canada had followed the model of Trudeau's Adirondack Cottage Sanitarium in Saranac Lake.

Dr. David C. Twitchell, an assistant resident physician at the sanitarium in 1903, writing in the Albuquerque *Morning Journal* called him "one of the leading figures in American medicine for the past twenty-five years" (Scrapbook 10, p. 8). While his clinical skills and method of treatment won Trudeau great recognition and gratitude from patients, his ingenuity as a researcher led to expressions of great respect from the scientists of his day.

Simon Flexner, professor at Johns Hopkins, praised him as "a great teacher in medicine. . . . Wherever the science of medicine is cultivated there is known Saranac Lake and Dr. Trudeau and his band of patient workers" (Scrapbook 10, p. 6). Celebrating the first twenty-five years of the Adirondack Cottage Sanitarium, Flexner had written, "The obvious element in Dr. Trudeau's professional life has been a high degree of sensitiveness to the impending great movements in medicine about to affect the problems of tuberculosis" (Flexner, 1910, p. 172). Coming from a noted medical scientist at one of the most respected medical schools in the country, these words were high praise. Sir William Osler, who left Johns Hopkins to teach at Oxford, praised Trudeau in the same 1910 edition:

The strong fibred nature of Trudeau is best illustrated by the fact that amid the worries of patients and the perennial financial struggle to make both ends meet he stuck close to the scientific side of his profession and from the laboratory of the Sanitarium have come many important contributions which have enriched the literature, and reflected the greatest credit upon American medicine (Osler, 1910, p. 163).

In Albany the *Knickerbocker Press* quoted Dr. Hermann M. Biggs, State Commissioner of Health, who said, "No one else in America has contributed as much as Dr. Trudeau to the direct solution of the practical problems of treatment or the elucidation of the scientific questions involved" (Scrapbook 10, p. 15). Biggs's contribution to the special edition of the *Journal of the Outdoor Life* credited Trudeau with a "fundamental change in the method of treatment of pulmonary tuberculosis," which led to "hundreds of clinics and sanatoria throughout the country":

Tens of thousands of persons owe their health and their lives to his strong and beneficent personality and the whole great movement here for the prevention and treatment of pulmonary tuberculosis may be said to have originated at Saranac Lake. . . .

The influence of Dr. Trudeau on the tuberculosis movement here and elsewhere is not wholly or even chiefly due to the results obtained in the Adirondack Cottage Sanitarium but rather to the high character of the scientific work which he has done, to the direct and indirect influence of his personality, to his unwavering enthusiasm and confidence and to his remarkable capacity for attracting, inspiring, and directing the work of his associates at Saranac Lake. Under his guidance there have been developed and trained at the Saranac Laboratory a group of men who have contributed many important publications on various phases of the tuberculosis problem and there have been sent out from this little village to various parts of the country numerous physicians and laymen full of Trudeau's beliefs and outlook as to the possibilities for the arrest and cure of this disease.

His personality and his scientific publications, together with those of the men whom he has directed and kept around him, . . . have made for the town of Saranac Lake a world wide reputation.

Every foreign scientist interested in the tuberculosis problem is perfectly familiar with the Adirondack Cottage Sanitarium and the work of the Saranac Laboratory, and its director (Biggs, 1910, p. 164).

Dr. Biggs, a renowned leader of the Public Health Movement in America, had worked with Trudeau organizing the National Association for the Study and Prevention of Tuberculosis; and Trudeau had supported Biggs's efforts to develop an effective bacteriological laboratory within the New York City Health Department. There were others who praised Dr. Trudeau in 1910 as well as after his death. Many were physicians who had come to the sanitarium to work as residents or to cure as patients. Others were patients who "cured" at the sanitarium or in the numerous cure cottages and summer homes throughout the area. Still others were local friends like Paul Smith (1910), the innkeeper who first introduced him to the Adirondacks, and Fitz Greene Halleck (1910), the local wilderness guide and woodsman who was a constant hunting and fishing companion.

The life and death of Edward Trudeau were felt by people from all levels of wealth, villagers from the Adirondack Mountains and residents of the largest cities, leaders of industry and business, and physicians and scientists of national and international reputations. What were the circumstances that led to this reputation? How could one health worker attract such universal recognition of his character, his clinical skills, his scientific acumen, and his leadership abilities? In the pages that follow I will try to answer these questions.

2

Trudeau's Early Life and Medical Training

Edward Trudeau was born into a heritage of medicine in 1848. His father was James de Berty Trudeau of New Orleans, an American physician and avid outdoorsman of French Huguenot descent. His mother, Céphise Berger, was the daughter of a prominent New York City physician and his equally prominent American wife Rebecca Aspinwall, daughter of a well-to-do merchant.

Trudeau's parents separated shortly after his birth. James, though he had been a founder of the prestigious New York Academy of Medicine, returned with Edward's older sister to New Orleans, where he alternated medical practice with naturalist scientific expeditions to the West. Around 1841 he spent two years living with the Osage Indians and later did the anatomy studies for several of J. J. Audubon's tours to the West. Until he was wounded he served as an officer in the Army of the Confederacy during the Civil War. Edward commented about his father, "The love of wild nature and of hunting was a real passion with my father—a passion which ruined his professional career in New Orleans, for he was constantly absent on hunting expeditions" (Trudeau, 1915, p. 10).

Céphise took her two sons to live with her father, Dr. François Eloi Berger, who retired from his practice in New York City and returned to his native Paris. From age three Edward Trudeau lived in Paris and attended the celebrated Lycée Bonaparte where his friends included Ned Dayton, son of the American ambassador. Although in later years Trudeau saw his French education as a negative experience—"the main idea was not to get caught"—he did read and speak French comfortably and was appreciative of European cosmopolitan ways (Trudeau, 1915, p. 15).

After the Civil War ended in 1865, the seventeen-year-old Edward and his older brother, Francis, returned to the United States to earn a living. Back in his native land he spoke English with a French accent. Because of his social class, family connections through his grandmother Aspinwall, and a small inheritance, he was not expected merely to get a job.

Trudeau was too well-connected for the vulgarities of trade or the vanities of public life. Although his trust fund was insufficient for more than clothes and spending money, he frequented the circles of his prosperous, socially prominent cousins the Livingstons, maintained membership in the Union Club, and cut a figure—a man about town, indistinguishable from dozens of other polished hedonists constitutionally incapable of earning a livelihood. Tall and spare, with aquiline features, muttonchop whiskers, and a somewhat prominent forehead, he took pains with creases and buttons, and might have stepped out of a novel of manners by Henry James or William Dean Howells, a young man of intelligence and breeding, unable to commit himself to an orthodox future (Taylor, 1986, p. 45).

While the enjoyable life of a tall, athletic bachelor appealed to the young Trudeau, reality confronted him early in September 1865, when his brother contracted tuberculosis and died in three months. Instead of entering the Naval Academy at Annapolis, Edward returned to New York City and cared for his brother. Much later, Trudeau remembered that the attending doctor had ordered the windows of Francis's stuffy room closed. Only toward the end, when his brother was gasping for air, was Edward allowed to open them.

Through one of his Aspinwall cousins, Trudeau met and fell in love with Charlotte Beare, daughter of an Episcopal rector in Little Neck, Long Island. Lottie supported this leaning toward the healing profession that Trudeau had so intimately experienced while caring for his brother. Having failed at several occupations and wanting to demonstrate to Miss Beare that he had a career worthy of her, Edward paid his five dollar admission fee and enrolled at the College of Physicians and Surgeons in the fall of 1868. His male cousins and friends at the Union Club predicted that he would never graduate. "The College of Physicians and Surgeons, on the corner of Twenty-third Street and Fourth Avenue, was a shabby brick building with a drugstore and an ice cream parlor tucked in the basement" (Taylor, 1986, p. 45). It would become part of Columbia University in 1891. We have this description of the school as it existed about 1872 shortly after Trudeau had graduated:

Physicians and Surgeons was the oldest and best and most arrogant of the three quarrelsome medical schools in New York City. The others were that of New York University—actually a proprietary school which bought diplomas from the University—and the Bellevue Hospital school. If the "University" and Bellevue schools were inferior to their great rival, this was not because Physicians and Surgeons had raised a standard to which the wise and foresighted could repair. It was a good school of a bad kind, a business enterprise with no admission requirements, an ungraded course, a single examination at the end of a man's studies, and a healthy respect for Gresham's law of proprietary schools—not to raise one's standards very far above the level of one's worst rival because there would be no standard to maintain if the students took their fees elsewhere (Fleming, 1987, p. 245).

Dr. T. Mitchell Prudden described the school in 1873, when no laboratory existed:

Pathological laboratories were rare in this country, and such as did exist were usually small corners in the "dead house" of some hospital. In the medical colleges . . . the student could, if he were enterprising, witness an occasional autopsy, but beyond this his knowledge of the fundamental theme was derived from lectures, charts, and books (Hotaling, 1991, p. 3, quoting Prudden, 1927).

From today's vantage point the school seems lacking, but it was the best available in New York City in 1868. The faculty of the college largely consisted of men from the thirty-four-member Medical and Surgical Society of New York and the 273-member New York Academy of Medicine (Rosenberg, 1967). Trudeau in his autobiography wrote:

The requirements for a medical student in those days were of the simplest. There was no entrance examination. All the student had to do was to matriculate at the college and pay a fee of five dollars, attend two or more courses of lectures at the college and pass the very brief oral examinations which each professor gave the members of the graduating class on his own subject. In addition, the law required that every student enter his name with some reputable practicing physician for three years as a student in his office—a rather hazy and indefinite relation, for which he paid the physician one hundred dollars each year. If those requirements were met the long-hoped for sheepskin was forthcoming and the new M.D. was turned loose on the world to meet as best he could the complicated responsibilities of a medical career (Trudeau, 1915, pp. 37–38).

Trudeau's intelligence and education had little to do with his matriculation, as the five-dollar fee was the only requirement. On the other hand, these qualities and his family may have helped him enlist Dr. Henry Sands, an eminent surgeon, as his preceptor and mentor. A church organist before becoming a physician, Dr. Sands taught surgery at Physicians and Surgeons and was an alumnus of the school. As a member of the New York Academy of Medicine he knew Edward's father and grandfather and was physician to the Livingston family. As a member of the New York Pathological Society and the Medical and Surgical Society he was part of an elite network of physicians. Serving as an attending surgeon at St. Luke's, Bellevue, and Roosevelt Hospitals in 1870, he could provide Trudeau with a wide range of clinical experiences.

With an inheritance of about $700 a year, augmented by another at his grandmother Aspinwall's death and later by funds from his grandfather's estate, Trudeau was able to attend one of the best medical schools in New York, maintain his friendships by taking meals at his club, and court Lottie, sometimes rowing his racing shell to her home on Long Island. In three years with his mentor, the young apprentice was introduced to the challenges and rewards of medicine in a large city. He aspired to a similar eminent career. He graduated in 1870 and took competitive exams for the position of house physician at the Stranger's Hospital, where Dr. Sands was in charge of surgery. He calculated that this was the most expedient way to finish his studies and achieve his major goal of marrying Lottie. At this time only about 20 percent of medical graduates did internships, which were not required. An even smaller proportion were able to study abroad (Hotaling, 1991, p. 4).

On January 1, 1871, Trudeau began six months of work at Stranger's, at the end of which he married Lottie on June 29, 1871. After a brief trip to the White Mountains in New England they sailed for Europe on the Cunarder *Russia,* returning in October on the *China.* Not only did they visit his remarried mother in Paris, but they saw Switzerland, Germany, and England as well.

THE SPECTRUM OF MEDICAL PRACTICES

What was the spectrum of medical practices in the early 1800s? Remembering that most people lived in rural areas and were largely dependent upon themselves for medical care, it is too simple to discuss the varieties of medical practices by using the major systems that attracted adherents, produced a body of literature, and created organizations. Eighteenth- and nineteenth-century archaeological evidence reveals an endless supply of medicines, sold over the counter or by itinerant peddlers, that were self-administered and then thrown into a privy or backyard dumping site (Blades, 1978; Haskell, 1981). Though the archaeological evidence contains only inert remains that were preserved, the organic remedies like mustard plasters and garlic cloves did not usually survive. In a time when most of the population was isolated on farms and in small hamlets, people gambled by treating themselves, passed down an oral tradition of family remedies, and relied on friends. Often they trusted clergymen, midwives, and people who called themselves physicians, but the variation must have been tremendous. Just as clergy attempted to define the limits of the faith, groups of physicians attempted to define the limits of their medical practice, including those of like belief and excluding all others. In the medicine of 1800, as in the religion of 1800, heresy was defined by groups of believers banding together to legitimate each other and exclude nonbelievers.

Although the full spectrum of medical practices awaits careful analyses of diaries and other material (Ulrich, 1990), several medical systems are usually discussed, reflecting some of the variety of formal medical thinking—allopathy,

Thomsonianism, homeopathy, and eclectics. While these categories formally order our thinking using data from written documents, the real picture must have shown considerably greater idiosyncratic variation.

Allopathic physicians were known in the early 1800s for their use of heroic treatments—"blood letting, blistering, leeching, cupping, sweating and purging"—with the wholesale use of calomel, a mercury compound used as a purgative, resulting in cathartic bowel movements (Kaufman, 1971, p. 100).

In contrast to the heroic methods of allopathic practitioners, the Thomsonians used natural remedies, which did considerably less physical harm. Because it was less violent, less expensive, and could be used by people isolated on their farms, Thomson's system raised a significant threat to allopathic practitioners and their livelihoods.

Homeopathy, a system imported from Germany, provided more competition for allopathic physicians. By administering infinitesimal amounts of a drug (1/500,000 to 1/1,000,000 of a grain) that at full strength produced the same symptoms as a disease, the homeopathic physician claimed to stimulate the vital forces within the body to fight the disease. The natural restorative powers of the body were further stimulated by "exercise, a nourishing diet, and pure air" (Kaufman, 1971, pp. 24–26). In a perfectionist religious climate this treatment had a certain logic and simplicity that attracted many patients.

By mid-century homeopathy had gained considerable stature. In the cholera epidemic of 1848 to 1852, homeopathic treatment "proved more effective than allopathic remedies." Public support for homeopaths was strong in states like Michigan. That state's legislature repealed medical licensing laws that allopathic physicians had supported to exclude homeopaths. Despite the allopaths' organized power base, by about 1870 homeopaths had won public and political support and formed their own medical society.

Eclecticism became a moderating influence among the rival systems. Eclectics strongly opposed the attempts by dogmatic allopathic practitioners to restrict medical practice. They advocated the novel idea that whatever helped the patient should be used regardless of the system.

With no standards or government controls defining what could be used as a medicine and a general desperation to find cures that actually worked, there was a free flow of ideas among individuals and the several organized medical groups. Allopathic physicians competed with Thomsonians, homeopaths, and eclectics in the free-wheeling Jacksonian era. The competition, clothed in the rhetoric of protecting the public from unqualified and poorly trained practitioners, was over control of the medical profession and the lucrative rewards to be gained therefrom.

The rivalry became politicized after allopathic physicians organized the American Medical Association in 1846. It established minimal educational standards for the medical degree and by 1855 demanded that "all state and local societies purge homeopaths from their ranks" (Kaufman, 1971, p. 55).

Its code of ethics contained the infamous "consultation clause," which stated that "No homeopath . . . could consult with an orthodox physician, even if the patient requested such a meeting. Likewise, no regular practitioner could come to the aid of a patient whose doctor was a homeopath, unless the homeopath was first dismissed from the case, regardless of how desperately ill the patient, or how necessary the consultation" (Kaufman, 1971, p. 53). We shall see how Edward Trudeau confronted this problem when asked to treat President Garfield's wife. By organizing medical societies, founding schools, publishing journals, and gaining popular support these groups developed enough political support, at least in the Northeast, to dominate the profession and control admission.

When Edward Trudeau began medical school in 1868 the American medical profession was on the brink of dramatic changes. Among a few scientists the germ theory of disease was just beginning its long journey to acceptance by the medical profession. Practitioners were often poorly trained, careless, unable to cure diseases, and helpless in the face of epidemics. The heterogeneous groups of allopaths, homeopaths, Thomsonians, and eclectics augmented by osteopaths, chiropractors, and Christian Scientists created an impossible puzzle for most citizens.

Physicians were helpless before diseases that they did not understand or treat with any predictable results. Some adopted rigid systems that they applied automatically to diseases they judged to be similar. Others followed the successes of their experience, using remedies passed down from previous generations, learned from native American healers, or stumbled across by chance.

A colonial practitioner's degree of success had been dependent on the degree of confidence he could inspire. But few could honestly claim an ability to cure certain types of disease consistently. Confidence was instead based on published or oral testimonials of occasional remarkable cures, which were often said to have been achieved through experience, a special knack, or divine inspiration (Kett, 1968, p. 178).

Dramatic social changes were sweeping the country. In 1800 most Americans lived in very small communities or on farms by themselves. By 1890, 37 percent lived in towns of 2,500 or more (Starr, 1982, p. 69). The growth of communities was primarily due to the migration of people from Europe and the British Isles attracted to industrial centers, creating the crowding and poverty that encouraged contagious diseases (Rosen, 1983, p. 37).

As people became concentrated in growing communities, physicians were less dispersed and more conscious of one another. Like-minded practitioners tended to band together, form associations, and develop the communities of common belief and practice that supported their own points of view. In some instances the boundaries between medical communities became so important that the welfare of the patient became secondary.

At the beginning of the nineteenth century the major killers of Americans were tuberculosis and the communicable diseases of childhood. In the larger cities tuberculosis was the leading cause of death. In New York City, for example, from 1804 to 1808 the tuberculosis death rate was 550 per 100,000 people (Lowell, 1969, p. 7). From 1811 to 1820, 6,061 or 23.4 percent of the 25,896 reported deaths were from tuberculosis (Waksman, 1964. p. 20, quoting Shattuck). By about 1840, rates for tuberculosis were near their peak, accounting for about 20 percent of all deaths (Long, 1956). In the period from 1849 to 1853 the city's death rate for tuberculosis had apparently decreased to 400 per 100,000 or about 11 percent of all deaths. In 1868, the year that Trudeau began his education, the rate was 533 per 100,000 New Yorkers (Waksman, 1964, p. 20, quoting Drolet, 1923). In the first half of the century, "the proportion of deaths ascribed to tuberculosis ranged from 15 to 30 percent" (Lowell, 1969, p. 7). By 1873 a decline had begun so that one in seven deaths, about 14 percent, was due to tuberculosis (Caldwell, 1988, p. 246). By the turn of the century, 1900–1904, "tuberculosis in the United States was causing 184.8 deaths per 100,000 people per year. This represented roughly 11 percent of all deaths at the time" (Caldwell, 1988, p. 247).

Figure 2.1
Death Rate for Tuberculosis, 1860–1960, United States

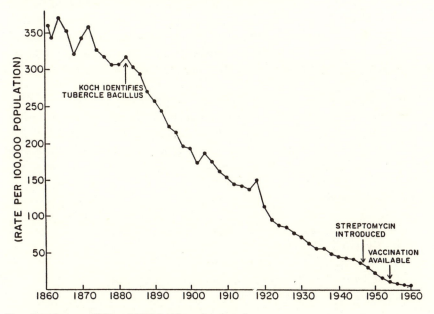

Note: Data between 1860 and 1900 for Massachusetts only.
Source: U.S. Bureau of the Census, *Historical Statistics of the United States: Colonial Times to 1970* (Washington, D.C.: Government Printing Office, 1975), Part 1, pp. 58, 63.

As people concentrated in the cities, infectious diseases could spread easily. Toward the end of the century health officials began to use public health methods and make some progress against "the white plague." The decline continued to an impressive low rate of 4.1 per 100,000 in 1963–67 (Spiegelman and Erhardt, 1974, p. 21). Only in the last decade has tuberculosis increased dramatically as cities and their inhabitants have again been neglected.

Encouraged by a Jacksonian political climate that allowed all medical systems complete freedom to compete for patients in the first half of the nineteenth century, the spectrum of medical practices was exceedingly broad and varied. "In the Jacksonian era, professional monopolies were assailed in the same spirit as business monopolies" (Starr, 1982, p. 140). One doctor's cure had as much legitimacy as another in the eyes of common citizens and politicians were reluctant to restrict the medical practices of one group in favor of another. By 1850, Lemuel Shattuck, a Boston merchant, "declared in his celebrated *Report of the Sanitary Commission of Massachusetts* that anyone, male or female, learned or ignorant, an honest man or a knave, can assume the name of physician and 'practice' upon anyone, to cure or to kill, as either may happen, without accountability. It's a free country!" (Kaufman, 1971, pp. 48–49).

Slowly the European laboratories and scientists who had trained some privileged Americans for about 100 years began to have greater influence. Their growing knowledge, facilitated by the development of scientific instruments, technology, and methods and fortified by support among the elite, became the basis for a new form of American medicine. A wave of change was just beginning to redesign most medical education in the country (Handlin, 1987, p. v–vi).

While their medical societies competed, some physicians began to place more emphasis on the role of clinical medicine in making therapeutic decisions (Warner, 1986, p. 52). Rather than follow a system and automatically bleed every feverish patient, doctors began to observe the effects of their ministrations and keep track of what produced positive results. They were following the method suggested by a Frenchman, Pierre Louis, who used a standard methodology for thoroughly studying each patient as he or she was being treated. By keeping detailed statistics on patients and doing autopsies on those who died, he based clinical investigation on data and gave more credence to clinical opinions. Eventually, allopathic physicians adopted ideas from the homeopaths and began to encourage the natural restorative powers of the body. "The relief of suffering rather than the active cure of disease, some physicians argued, was their principal task" (Warner, 1986, p. 97). Building up the natural restorative powers of the body became a generally accepted goal for most physicians.

In the second half of the 1800s new instruments and devices allowed medical practitioners to see and hear signs in forms that appeared to be objective.

Trudeau was not trained to use a microscope in medical school. The device was perfected in Europe to the extent that Rudolph Virchow published *Cellular Pathology* in 1858, describing microscopic changes in normal cells produced by disease processes and making "the cell the ultimate morphological unit within which life could exist" (Reiser, 1978, p. 78). Microscopy stimulated the development of bacteriology, allowing the French chemist Louis Pasteur to prove that the decay of organic matter always occurred in the presence of microorganisms. By 1870 Pasteur was warning surgeons to sterilize their hands and clean their instruments with boiling water and flame. Joseph Lister, an English surgeon, used this knowledge to prevent infection of surgical wounds by destroying bacteria with chemical antiseptics like carbolic and phenic acid (Reiser, 1978, p. 83). At this time, just before the germ theory was to gain wide acceptance, Edward Trudeau began his medical career.

Although the formality of medical school lectures precluded seeing patients, Trudeau's apprenticeship to Dr. Henry Sands and his internship at Stranger's Hospital must have given him experience with the stethoscope, which had become an accepted tool for examining patients by 1850 (Reiser, 1978, p. 38).

Just as Trudeau began studying, a German physician, Carl Wunderlich, published *On the Temperature in Diseases*, describing temperature variations in thirty-two common diseases. The thermometer became another tool that signified an educated physician and gave numerical evidence of the febrile condition that had been recognized for centuries.

The new science of chemistry was applied to the analysis of body fluids like blood and urine so that they could be described in their normal and diseased states. Laboratories did not exist in American medical schools in 1868 and Trudeau was not taught chemistry, but these skills represented the direction in which medical science was going.

During the period that Trudeau was trained, the identity and status of the physician were changing. His teachers depended upon their ability to create an "aura of certitude" by gentlemanly dress, etiquette, demeanor, and good judgment. Trudeau's generation would be judged by these things but also upon their acquaintance with the latest knowledge, their mastery of the latest technologies, and their ability to apply that knowledge successfully to patients. The control that had come from heroic procedures early in the century and from pharmaceuticals after mid-century was beginning to be maintained by letting "science decide the most prudent course."

WHAT TRUDEAU LEARNED

By the time Trudeau entered medical school, three main currents of medical thinking were popular among the public and commonly followed by New York City practitioners.

1. Nature provided better medical care than the prevailing system (Kaufman, 1971, p. 33). This faith in the curative power of nature was a contribution of homeopathy.

2. Hahnemann's "experimental pharmacology" provided the basis for "careful observation of effects of specific remedies" and established a body of knowledge related to these effects, which could be taught and learned (Kett, 1965, p. 163).

3. The interests of the patient began to take precedence over sectarian medical interests. This led to abandoning the "consultation clause" of the American Medical Association (allopaths) because "an increasing number of physicians had become convinced that homeopaths were well educated men trying to minister to the sick" (Kaufman, 1971, p. 127).

It is safe to assume that these ideas existed at the College of Physicians and Surgeons, but whether they were dominant or not is unclear. The allopathic medicine that Trudeau learned in 1868–70 had been changed by competition with other systems over several decades.

Heroic methods had not completely disappeared. Throughout the handwritten notes taken by several students on the lectures of Trudeau's professor, Alonzo Clark, there are numerous references to venesection for meningitis (Hutchison, 1865–66, pp. 20–21) and pneumonia (Dodge, 1867–78, no pages). [Quotes from these notes will include errors. My additions will be in brackets.] Clark recommended bleeding the young by applying leeches. Older patients were "bled while sitting up in bed until face becomes pale and perspiration stands on his forehead" (Hutchison, 1865–66, pp. 20–21). Also, in those days Clark used calomel (mercurous chloride), a purgative or cathartic that could cause rather profound bowel movements depending upon the dosage (Dodge, 1867–68, no pages). But such heroic methods were not suggested for tuberculosis.

In his autobiography Trudeau related what his professor taught about tuberculosis:

Dr. Alonzo Clark taught that it was a non-contagious, generally incurable and inherited disease, due to inherited constitutional peculiarities, perverted humors and various types of inflammation, and dwelt at length on the different pathological characteristics of tubercle, scrofula, caseation, and pulmonary phthisis, and their classification and relation to each other (Trudeau, 1915, pp. 40–41).

Clark's ideas about tuberculosis can be expanded by quoting from a speech to the New York State Medical Society and members of the legislature in February 1853, in which he sought to enlighten legislators about conditions affecting health in New York City. "We hear enumerated among the causes of tubercular consumption, imperfect protection either by house or clothing, against the vicissitudes of weather; scanty and unnutritious food; imperfect ventilation, vitiated air; dwelling in dark, damp places; indifference to personal cleanliness—if society has improved in these then tuberculosis should recede" (Clark, 1853, p. 19).

The Frenchman, J. A. Villemin had been able to convey tuberculosis from man to animals in 1865. After this demonstration European physicians began to believe that tuberculosis was contagious. It was recognized as a specific disease that could be prevented by "the improvement of habitations and working conditions, the maintenance of a high standard of health, and, if possible, a return to the practice of disinfection of things and places that have been contaminated by consumptives" (Waksman, 1964, p. 84). By the time that Trudeau entered medical school at least some Europeans were convinced that tuberculosis was contagious, but on the other side of the Atlantic the chairman of medicine at the College of Physicians and Surgeons taught an older idea. Tuberculosis was contracted by people who were exposed to "certain disease-inducing 'miasmatic' conditions in the environment" (Cooter, 1982, p. 94). As far as Clark was concerned it was best to avoid these conditions as much as possible. Perhaps the best statement of Alonzo Clark's position comes from hand written notes of his lectures by Dr. A. R. M. Purdy, an 1861 graduate of the college. Purdy lists as some of the most prominent causes of tuberculosis:

1st Hereditary predisposition must be regarded foremost of all these. Then again it may not appear in the parent as a disease, but the children may have it in consequence of degeneration, owing to close intermarriage, such as cousin to cousin, etc.

2nd Climate is of great importance in producing this disease. Temperate regions are the most liable. Damp cold winds seem to have a very decided influence in producing it. Statistics show that those counties along the New England coast (Essex, Cape Cod, etc.) which are constantly subjected to the influence of the winds blowing from Newfoundland, have the mortality greatly increased in comparison with those further inland, like Berkshire.

3rd Poverty: living in cold, dark, damp cellars; bad food, etc. is another cause. Dark damp places exert a bad influence. Insufficient food also acts unfavorably.

These then are some of the most important circumstances that tend to produce the disease (Purdy, 1890, p. 90, second book).

In this lecture and in Clark's address to the state legislators can be seen the seeds of public health physicians' concerns about poverty, filth, and poor living conditions. Clark's lecture went on to talk about treatment:

The first question is: Is consumption curable? I put my faith in the doctrine that it is. I know that I have seen 100 cases that have been cured under my own personal observation.

In attempting a cure of this disease. Your object is to prevent the deposit of more tubercules. You cannot stop the course of those already begun (Purdy, 1890, p. 90 second book).

The idea that tuberculosis was curable must have come as a surprise to Trudeau, who had experienced the death of his brother and probably accepted the prevailing idea that consumption was usually fatal. In fact, he noted in his biography that Clark had taught that it was "non-contagious, generally incurable and inherited." Presumably, Trudeau and his fellow students had seen tubercles, these small rounded nodules, in *Gray's Anatomy* or on the lungs of a cadaver in the dissecting room on the top floor of the college. This translucent mass of gray spherical cells or a yellowish mass of cheesy matter was the characteristic lesion [abnormality] observed on the lungs of those who died from pulmonary consumption.

Clark would then describe the following treatment:

We have known that where there is a loss of vitality, there is the danger of the tuberculous deposit.

Assuming then, that this doctrine is correct, the first thing that would suggest itself is to build up. Give the best food: best mutton, best beef, anything and everything substantial; Porter wine and even brandy for the same purpose. But in administering liquors, you must have moderation, always stopping short of the nervous influences it produces. The patient must never feel it in the head; for any excess in liquor, as is well known, predisposes to tuberculous disease.

Resort to the best use of external air. Whenever it is warm and bland and if it be a man who is tolerably strong, let him go out in all weathers, and walk a mile or so.

Next, keep the functions of the skin in good condition by bathing and active friction. You can use cold or tepid sponging in the morning followed by friction and warm friction before going to bed.

In regard to the bowels, you generally will have very little trouble until the diarrhea occurs. If they will not act right, give an enema of cold water or a Blue pill will answer.

If the appetite be not good: use Stomachics as Tinct. Gentian, Strenglitron's bitters, Tansy and wine and other bitter tonics an hour or so before eating. The chief of these means is exercise in the open air.

But stop, are you not going to give medication in any form? Yes, give Cod liver oil. I recommend its use with my whole heart. It is the only medicine that has held its ground after a trial of 40 years, and seems to increase in favor year after year. It is given in dessert spoonful doses. But inasmuch as the oil is so disagreeable to some, I think you can use in place of that, and with all its advantages, the cream of milk; half a pint or more after each meal. Or you may give olive oil mixed with iodine. I have found it to answer an excellent purpose . . . I have found it equally good as Cod Liver Oil.

In fact, we can use any oil. It is an important element in the organization of the tissues, and by forcing on the system an extra quantity of fat, you force the system to take it up.

I think the theory that I have adopted (though I can't prove a word of it) holds out best in connection with the standard principles of treatment (Purdy, 1890, pp. 90–92, second book).

The goal of this treatment was to build up the body so that it could restore itself. This was called "the general treatment," emphasizing that its goal was to improve the general health of the patient so that the body's natural healing processes could restore health. By the 1880s allopathic medicine had adopted this idea from homeopathy, and Trudeau accepted it.

Clark gave suggestions to his students for treating the various symptoms associated with tuberculosis.

The first condition I shall notice is *Cough*. Now I advise you not to give much medicine for the cough. Just recollect that the patient must cough and will cough. And if you stop the cough, you stop the expectoration and as it were, drown the patient in his own fluids. If the cough be light, you resort to syrups or candy which excite the secretions first in the mouth, and so for a certain extent in the Bronchial tubes.

If the cough throws off sufficiently let it alone: only interfere when the cough is excessive and the expectorations small. You may also use Balsam Tolu 4 to 5 dropped into syrup of Ipecac. This will tend to check the secretion when too large. Opium allays the nervous irritability. If there be a dry wheezing cough coming on in paroxysms and annoying the patient by its frequency, and force, then you are justified in interfering, and trying to relieve him. For this purpose you have a vast number of cough medicines and those which are most efficacious contain opium in some of its forms. Besides opium, prussic acid has sometimes been given with advantage. If there be any considerable amount of inflammatory complication. I suppose you would with propriety enough give Tart. Eruetic, but I would not use it often, and I would not use it at all if the pulse is any way excited. The syrup of Prunus Virginiana is a very excellent medicine, particularly, if combined with a small quantity of Morphine: it is both soothing and tonic in its character and I have known it to give tone to the stomach when nothing else would. I have used when the patient has considerable strength, Ayers Cherry Pectoral, quack medicine though it be and I have found it to answer a very good purpose. I give it because I know its composition. It is not applicable when the patient is prostrated as it contains tartar of antimony. But in the main, I think you can place the best reliance on the general treatment.

Next, in regard to Haemoptysis [coughing blood]. The first thing you are called to do, when it occurs, is to quiet your patient's fears. Of course, you must not ridicule their ideas, but make light of it. Kindly persuade them that it is of no consequence. You can appreciate the importance of this when you recollect the influence excitement has in keeping up the action of the heart; and to keep down his apprehensions you can give some medicine to give him the idea that you are doing something for it. Give anything you like, any placebo will do: a little dose of salt and water. If the hemorrhage is any way profuse, you can give rousing doses of opium (2 to 3 grs). Keep him quiet and in bed in any case. Keep his head elevated and keep him in a cool place: not so cold as to excite bleeding. I would not bleed as a general rule: only in those cases where there is a good deal of vigor in the system, and plethora, and then blood must be taken and cleanly and by a rousing stream = about 6 oz. Otherwise it will do mischief. If you take too much blood, it loses its coagulability, and the hemorrhage is difficult to stop. In that profuse hemorrhage that is consequent upon the [unreadable] of a vessel, your patient faints as a general rule pretty early and by the syncope, a clot is formed in the cavity which plugs up the vessel; and you have two things to look out for: 1st not to arouse him too soon from the syncope and 2nd not to leave him too long in it.

Next of the night sweats. These generally occur about the middle stage of the disease, sometimes at the first stage and then reappear at the latter part. In regard to the care of these, in the majority of cases I don't think you can do anything. When the chill comes on in the morning you can treat it the same as an intermittent with your Quinine and Excess of Elixir of Vitriol. If the sweats occur at night you may adopt the same plan, only perhaps upon a milder principle. Dr. Gilman's "pickled towels" are very good here again, frictions with alcohol, Tincture of pepper, etc. are very serviceable, or Alum and Alcohol. If the sweating greatly weakens you may give Acid. Sulph, as a tonic, or combined with Quinine and the Sulphate of Quinine.

One word about the voice, when in the milder, or early stages of the disease you can accomplish a great deal by the direct applications of Nit. Arg. (in solution) or a sponge, squeezing it against the opening, and allowing a few drops to go into the larynic, and upon the vocal cords. But in the latter periods of the disease, your main reliance must be upon the general treatment for the disease in the Lungs.

Yes Gentlemen, I believe this seems to be the whole thing. You observe the upshot of the matter is that your general treatment is the thing for all: it is that which is to cure all these symptoms and diminish your special prescriptions as much as possible (Purdy, 1890, pp. 2–94, second book).

When one of Trudeau's fellow students developed symptoms similar to those of his brother, Trudeau presented his friend's case to Dr. Clark and received this brief advice about treatment: "Tell your friend to go to the mountains and become a stage driver for a few years" (Trudeau, 1915, p. 41).

It was this knowledge that Trudeau was given at medical school. When he worked at the Stranger's Hospital he acquired valuable experience. At Bellevue Clinic, Dr. Austin Flint, one of his medical professors, and Dr. Edward Janeway praised Trudeau's ability to diagnose tuberculosis in its early stages (Harrod, 1959, p. 62). Appointment at a hospital allowed Trudeau to develop experience with pulmonary disease, giving him some skill and standing as a specialist compared to general practitioners. Such temporary hospital appointments often led to an appointment with full attending privileges in a hospital (Rosen, 1983, p. 33). Trudeau was well situated to begin a promising medical career. Whether he had accepted the European idea that tuberculosis was contagious is unknown.

This was the professional input to Trudeau's knowledge of tuberculosis by 1872. Probably from caring for his brother in 1865, Trudeau had acquired tuberculosis himself. As a result he was to gain a more intimate and existential understanding of the disease. While he suffered the life of a tuberculosis invalid first hand he did not spend much time reading the medical literature on tuberculosis for about seven years.

3

Trudeau's Personal Experience with Tuberculosis

Caring for his brother during the last three months of 1865, living in the same room and often sharing the same bed, exposed the unsuspecting Trudeau to tuberculosis bacilli. The New York City environment of those days was not a healthy place, and tuberculosis was endemic. Crammed into the southern half of Manhattan were more than 650,000 people. The mortality rate of New York City was greater than that of Paris or London. Less than half of the homes or tenements had bathing facilities. Food was not fresh or clean. Physicians treated acute infectious diseases daily and were in intimate contact with their germs (Rosenberg, 1967). As a healthy young man he had been able to fight the disease, but the rigors of medical studies and an active social life began to have an effect. Sometime during the winter of 1869–70 friends at the Union Club wagered that he could walk from Central Park to the Battery in less than an hour. Wanting to please his friends Lou and Jim Livingston, Trudeau managed the walk in forty-seven minutes but felt ill long after (Trudeau, 1915, p. 51). Much later he consulted a doctor, who discovered a localized collection of pus in a cavity, forming a cold abscess that had to be drained several times before it healed. Trudeau commented, "In those days the relation of such cold abscesses to tuberculosis was not understood, and no one even hinted to me that it was of the least importance" (Trudeau, 1915, p. 51).

The next indication of the disease occurred during Edward and Lottie's honeymoon trip to Europe, June to October 1871. While they were in England Dr. Trudeau experienced "swelling of the lymphatic glands on the side of my neck, but so ignorant were we about the mechanism of tuberculous infection at that time that this symptom gave me no alarm" (Trudeau, 1915, p. 68). An

English physician in Liverpool examined him and concluded, "The glands were an evidence of a run-down condition and a tendency to scrofula; [he] advised me to paint them with iodine, eat plenty of bacon at my breakfast, and gave me a tonic with iron in it. This second warning of the tuberculous infection went as unheeded as the first, and I never realized that I was already infected with the disease that had run so rapid and fatal a course in my brother's case" (Trudeau, 1915, pp. 68–69).

Returning to the United States, Lottie and Edward settled into a cottage at the gate of W. P. Douglas's estate in Little Neck. By caring for local people and supplementing their income with their inheritance they lived quite comfortably. Edward had met Douglas when he crewed on Douglas's yacht *Sappho* in the America Cup race against the *Cambria* from England. Despite their comfortable situation, Trudeau was soon bored by a country practice and frustrated by isolation from medical colleagues and hospital work. In the fall of 1872 they moved to New York City, where he became a partner of Dr. Fessenden Otis, a professor of venereal and genito-urinary diseases at the College of Physicians and Surgeons and attending physician at Stranger's Hospital. Trudeau gradually replaced Otis on an increasing proportion of house calls (three to six a day), splitting the fee.

This return to the city connected Trudeau with established physicians (as Otis also belonged to the New York Academy of Medicine) who evidently respected him and allowed him to teach a class for diseases of the chest at the Demilt Dispensary with his fellow student Dr. Luis P. Walton. Together they examined and prescribed for patients for two hours, three times a week, treating charity patients in clinics at the hospital (Trudeau, 1915, p. 70).

During their year at Little Neck, Trudeau experienced "two or three . . . attacks of fever" but presumed it was malaria, as nearly everyone had it. He took quinine, which had no effect. After moving to New York Trudeau "felt tired all the time, but thought it was the confinement of city life and paid but little attention to it" (Trudeau, 1915, p. 70). Finally Dr. Walton "insisted that I looked ill and took my temperature." The discovery of a temperature of 101 degrees astonished Trudeau and worried him enough to take Walton's suggestion that he see Dr. Edward Janeway, whose physical diagnosis class at Bellevue Hospital he had attended.[1] Trudeau received the grave news that "the upper two-thirds of the left lung was involved in an active tuberculous process" (Trudeau, 1915, p. 71).

His reaction to this news tells us a lot about how he perceived tuberculosis as a disease in 1872 and what it meant to his professional ambitions.

I think I know something of the feeling of the man at the bar who is told he is to be hanged on a given date, for in those days pulmonary consumption was considered as absolutely fatal. . . . I had consumption—that most fatal of diseases! Had I not seen it in all its horrors in my brother's case? It meant death and I had never thought of death before! Was I ready to die? How could I tell my wife, whom I had just left in unconscious happiness with the little baby in our new home? And my rose-colored dreams of achievement and professional success in New York! They were all shattered now, and in their place only exile and the inevitable end remained! (Trudeau, 1915, pp. 71–72).

Convinced in his own mind that he was fatally ill and supported by his again pregnant wife, they left in a few days for Aiken, South Carolina, in February 1873. Trudeau was "told to live out of doors and ride on horseback" (the Syndenham treatment). This regular exercise resulted in the development of daily fever, and he had not improved upon returning to New York in April. Trudeau commented about this method of treatment: "I was allowed and even urged to exercise daily, in the misguided belief that it would improve my appetite and keep me from losing strength; but the result naturally enough was that my fever kept up and that I lost weight and strength steadily" (Trudeau, 1915, p. 73).

Assuming he was hopelessly ill, Trudeau gave up work and waited until Lottie delivered their son, Ned, on May 18, 1873. A week later, accompanied by Lou Livingston, he traveled to the Adirondack Mountains, a place he had visited two years earlier. Lottie returned with the two children to Little Neck to live with her father. Writing forty years later Trudeau revealed his frame of mind in making this trip:

I was influenced in my choice of the Adirondacks only by my love for the great forest and the wild life, and not at all because I thought the climate would be beneficial in any way, for the Adirondacks were then visited only by hunters and fishermen and it was looked upon as a rough, inaccessible region and considered a most inclement and trying climate. I had been to Paul Smith's in the summer on two occasions before on short visits with my friend Lou Livingston and his mother, and had been greatly attracted by the beautiful lakes, the great forest, the hunting and fishing, and the novelty of the free and wild life there. If I had but a short time to live, I yearned for surroundings that appealed to me, and it seemed to meet a longing I had for rest and the peace of the great wilderness (Trudeau, 1915, pp. 77–78).

The trip to Paul Smith's summer hotel was not easy. The first day was a long train ride from New York to Saratoga, a popular summer spa. Resting overnight, they continued by train to Whitehall at the southern tip of Lake Champlain, where they boarded a boat for Plattsburgh arriving for the evening meal. These two days made Trudeau so sick with a "raging fever" that he stayed in bed at the Fouquet House for the next two days. The hotel staff, fearing he would die, urged his friend Livingston to turn around and take Trudeau home. Nevertheless, on the fifth day they took another train to Ausable Forks and hired a two-horse stage. With Trudeau on a mattress between the two seats, they drove the forty-two mile corduroy road to Paul Smith's. The last day of the trip must have been very trying. He commented: "I stood the jolting pretty well until afternoon, when the fever and the fatigue made the rough shaking of the wagon almost unbearable" (Trudeau, 1915, p. 79). Though six feet three inches tall and athletic, his diseased body was so weak and frail that he had to be carried up two flights of stairs to his room by Fred Martin, a sturdy Adirondack guide.

Putting him down on the bed Fred Martin cracked:
"Why, Doctor, you don't weigh no more than a dried lamb-skin!" We both laughed, and indeed I was so happy at reaching my destination and seeing the beautiful lake again, the mountains and the forests all around me, that I could hardly have been depressed by anything Fred Martin could have said. During the entire journey I had felt gloomy forebodings as to the hopelessness of my case, but, under the magic influence of the surroundings I had longed for, these all disappeared and I felt convinced I was going to recover. How little I knew, as I shook hands with the great, strong men who came up to my room that evening to say a word of cheer to me, that forty-two years later most of them would be dead and that I should still be in the Adirondacks and trying to describe my first arrival at Paul Smith's as an invalid! Soon Katie Martin, Mrs. Paul Smith's pretty sister, came in with a word of welcome and cheer and a tray on which were eggs, brook trout, pancakes and coffee, and I ate heartily and with a real relish for the first time in many a long week (Trudeau, 1915, pp. 80–81).

Though Paul Smith's hotel lacked running water, it was clean and comfortable and had excellent food and warm, caring people. This produced a dramatic change in Trudeau's outlook, rid him of hopelessness, and created a renewed will to live. In this frame of mind and physically exhausted he slept very well and woke eager to enjoy his new surroundings. On his first day Warren Flanders, a guide, persuaded him to go out in a boat, reclining on blankets over balsam boughs. The beauty of the day and his surroundings lifted his spirits. He shot a deer and returned to the hotel triumphant (Trudeau, 1915, pp. 87–88). For someone who enjoyed all of wild nature, this must have been a tremendous source of pride and encouragement.

Trudeau's friend Lou Livingston stayed through July and was replaced by another friend, E. H. Harriman, in August and by Jim Livingston in September. By the end of September Trudeau had gained fifteen pounds and felt that his health had returned to normal. But the fever reappeared soon after his return to the city. His medical advisors suggested that the family winter in St. Paul, Minnesota, because its high proportion of sunny days was thought to be good for pulmonary invalids. Trudeau was allowed to drive a buggy, walk, and hunt ducks; by spring he was "nearly as sick as the year before and the Adirondacks seemed my only hope; so we left St. Paul in May, and early in June, accompanied by my wife, and two children and two nurses, I arrived at Paul Smith's to my intense joy, for I always loved the place" (Trudeau, 1915, p. 97).

During that summer of 1874, Trudeau did not improve. He consulted a summer resident, Dr. Alfred Loomis, a recovered consumptive, who confirmed Trudeau's continued tuberculous condition and agreed (as Loomis held no hope for recovery) with Trudeau's desire to avoid additional moves and take his chances by staying in the Adirondacks. (Loomis's article in the *Medical Record* says he "advised" Trudeau to spend the winter.) Having followed the best medical advice and gone to a warm climate in the winter of 1873, Trudeau was willing to gamble on the cold and storms of an Adirondack winter a year later, despite his colleagues' predictions that such an act "seemed to them little short of suicide" (Trudeau, 1915, p. 101). Much persuasion by Edward was required to convince the Paul Smith's staff that the Trudeaus should stay at the hotel beyond its normal closing date at the end of hunting season in October. The family spent the Adirondack winter sixty miles from the railroad and the closest doctor at Plattsburgh. They were isolated from the outside world except for a telegraph line and mail, which came by sleigh three times a week when the road was open.

Although Trudeau tried to be active and enjoyed hunting, he noticed that after walking he felt sick and feverish the next day, "and this was the first intimation I had as to the value of the rest cure, which in after years I applied so thoroughly and rigidly to my patients. I walked very little after this, and my faith in the value of the rest cure became more and more fully established" (Trudeau, 1915, pp. 107–108).

From his own experience Trudeau had discovered the connection between activity and fever for consumptives and the healing significance of complete rest. The result of that winter was that he felt somewhat better, and by the summer of 1875 he began to take an interest in his profession. He had given some medical aid to the occasional injured guide. That summer he ordered a supply of medicines and provided care to summer guests at Paul Smith's hotel.

When Alfred Loomis returned for his hunting trip in the fall of 1875, he examined Trudeau and found him no worse than the previous year. Surprised that Trudeau had survived at all, Loomis agreed to another winter. Unable to stay at Paul Smith's, the Trudeaus rented a small house in the village of Saranac Lake and spent the winter.

Trudeau began to gain weight and strength. Feeling better, he expanded his practice at Paul Smith's and other summer hotels as well as among the local people. Trudeau's tuberculosis was intermittent, and he learned to live with it, cutting back when the fever appeared, resting when the fatigue became intolerable. Whenever his health became poor, Trudeau credited retreat to his beloved woods and lakes as essential for his recovery. He wrote: "It is curious that this passion for the wild out-of-doors existence which wrecked my father's professional career, saved my life by enabling me to live contentedly in a wilderness during the first five years of my illness just the sort of life that was best adapted for my restoration to health" (Trudeau, 1915, pp. 10–11).

By 1876 Trudeau had decided that if he wanted to remain reasonably healthy he must deny his aspiration to become a prominent physician in New York City and develop a life in the most rural area of the Adirondack Mountains. Resigned to living away from his beloved city, Trudeau decided to make the best of his condition. As his health improved he began to participate in the community, to build a practice, especially among wealthy summer visitors from eastern cities, and to renew his connections with professional colleagues. Through his own personal experience with tuberculosis, he had been taught by the local guides a way he could survive the disease and stay alive. He drew upon this experience to develop a method of treating patients that brought him considerable recognition and esteem from the public and his professional peers as well.

NOTE

1. Janeway, as curator at Bellevue Hospital, had been one of the first physicians to conduct systematic autopsies in New York City. He made pathological anatomy the basis for clinical diagnosis. When Trudeau consulted him in 1872, he had just become Professor of Pathological Anatomy at Bellevue Hospital Medical College. In 1875, Janeway became Commissioner of Health in New York City, where he advocated sanitation and preventive health measures. In 1892 he advised the New York Chamber of Commerce on ways to prevent an epidemic of cholera and was largely successful. The last twenty years of his life were spent as a consultant to all classes of patients because his charges were so modest. As an elder in the Dutch Reformed Church, he argued "that a consultant who accepts no patients except for opinion and advice to their physician occupies a stronger ethical position than one who may be persuaded to retain a wealthy patient for treatment." Dr. Janeway served as vice president of the New York Pathological Society and as president of the New York Academy of Medicine, the Association of American Physicians, and the National Association for the Study and Prevention of Tuberculosis. In all of these associations, Trudeau would participate.

4

Changing Knowledge of Tuberculosis in the Nineteenth Century

In the early nineteenth century tuberculosis killed proportionally more people than heart disease and cancer combined today. The "white plague" was considered absolutely fatal, an insidious disease that "consumed" its victims—thus the name "consumption." What caused tuberculosis was a mystery until 1882, but throughout the nineteenth century causal explanations changed as people learned more about the disease.

As early as 1685, it was known that many diseases produced "generalized emaciation" or "wasting," such as "severe diarrhea . . . , long continued blood loss, diabetes, dropsy, and chronic weeping ulcerations" (King, 1982, p. 18). Richard Morton (1635–1698) wrote *Phithisiologia: or a Treatise of Consumptions* in Latin, differentiating these generalized diseases from "consumption" or "phthisis," which he defined as a disease of the lungs. According to Morton, a case of pulmonary consumption could be distinguished by the following: "a wasting of the whole body (in contrast to a merely localized atrophy), a hectic fever, and an 'exulceration' of the lungs. This referred to the cough that at first was dry and nonproductive but later would become purulent—i.e., productive—and resulted in cavities in the lung" (King, 1982, p. 19). Because the condition of the blood was "sharp" and heated, causing inflammation,

the physician should temper the heat of the blood through gentle laxatives that will "carry off the load of humors by stool gently, and by degrees." Similarly in the early stage of the disease a moderate amount of blood-letting may "cool" the blood. An opiate will "quiet the lungs, which at this time are heated by the continual and violent motion of the cough," and also "calm the whole mass of blood" (King, 1982, p. 23).

Seventy-five years later, William Cullen (1710–1790) defined what he called "phthisis pulmonaris" as "an expectoration of pus or purulent matter from the lungs, attended with a hectic fever" (King, 1982, p. 26). Attention to this symptom allowed diagnosis before emaciation had actually occurred. By observing the color and odor of the sputum and noting whether it sank in water as well as its reactions to acids and alkalis, the physician could develop evidence to help him make a diagnosis. "Hectic fever" had special characteristics, "occurring in the morning and again in the evening, with more or less remission in between," and accompanied by a "febrile flush that mantled the cheeks during the exacerbations." Cullen noted that certain occupational groups who worked in dust such as "stone-cutters," were especially susceptible to "phthisis pulmonaris" (King, 1982, p. 27).

Autopsies had provided confirmation that the lungs were involved in consumption or phthisis and that the tubercle was related to the ulcerated growth. The process of tuberculosis was described in 1810 by a French physician Gaspard-Laurent Bayle (1774–1816). As soon as the first tubercle could be observed in the lung, before a cough or fever, the disease process had begun. Bayle argued that even though an early symptom might be "trivial, scarcely more than a slight indisposition, . . . it can progress to a massive ailment" (King 1982, p. 82). The idea that consumption was a progressive disease was very important.

At about this time Jean Nicolas Corvisart (1755–1821), another Frenchman, popularized the use of percussion—Auenbrugger's technique of tapping the chest and back to learn the condition of the lungs by the resultant sound. This allowed the identification of the diseased lung by comparing the sound to healthy lung sounds. Shortly afterward Rene Theopile-Hyacinthe Laennec (1787–1826) discovered that he could hear these sounds better by rolling paper into a cylinder and placing one end on the patient and the other to his ear. By 1819 he had developed the stethoscope into a wooden cylinder with a funnel-shaped hollow and published *On Mediate Auscultation.* Using this device Laennec "examined the character of sounds emanating from the chests of healthy and of ill patients, most of which he could relate to anatomical faults he found by dissecting their bodies after death" (Reiser, 1978, p. 25). For example, in 1821, in *A Treatise on the Diseases of the Chest* he stated that he had "not met with a single instance in which ulcerous excavations did not exist in those points of the lung over which the phenomenon of pectoriloquism had shown itself distinctly" (Reiser, 1978, p. 30, quoting Laennec's *Diseases of the Chest*). Laennec's precision was evident in his differentiation of phthisis or tuberculous phthisis from "lung abscess, anthracosis (coal miner's disease), or cancer." For him, phthisis was "the specific destructive disease of the lung uniquely associated with the tubercle, and the equivalent of what we now call pulmonary tuberculosis" (King, 1982, p. 35). Because Laennec died of tuberculosis in 1826, it was left to others to convince physicians of the usefulness of "mediate auscultation" (listening with the assistance of a stethoscope) in the diagnosis of consumption. As patients did not always report their symptoms accurately, physicians were urged to listen to patients' chests for themselves. Those who doubted the value of auscultation sought proof.

In the late 1820s when one physician, unconvinced of the superiority of physical diagnosis, challenged an auscultator, Dr. James Hope, to test the matter, a public trial of the old and new schools of diagnosis ensued. At St. George's Hospital, London, each physician examined the same patient, and each applied only his own techniques. Autopsy subsequently affirmed the correctness of the auscultator's diagnosis, and silenced the critic (Reiser, 1978, p. 31).

While the stethoscope sharpened the diagnosis of tuberculosis, it did nothing for the treatment.
    Autopsies revealed that the tubercle was always connected to the disease, but it was mid-century before the techniques of microscopy were sophisticated enough to begin to understand this structure. Microscopic examination

paid special attention to the granular substance of cheesy appearance, found in consumption. This matter, at first called "tuberculous matter," might appear in minute amounts in the center of a barely visible tubercle, or it might exist in massive quantities in lungs or lymph nodes. . . . The term "tubercle" acquired a dual meaning—the discrete small nodule and also the granular caseous [cheesy] matter. When the caseous substance was in question, the word "tubercle" was used in a generic sense, without any qualifying article. When, however, a discrete nodule was in question, pathologists spoke of "a" or "the" tubercle or, as with Virchow, a "true" tubercle. But "tubercle," unqualified, usually referred to caseous material as a general class (King, 1982, p. 46).

This tubercle, or "granular substance of cheesy appearance," characteristic of tuberculosis was produced, according to the blastema theory, when the blaste-mas from the blood produced cells that were tuberculous.

The blastemas, as a deposit or exudate, had varying potentialities to produce cells. There were three major types of exudate: inflammatory, cancerous, and tuberculous. Once these entered the tissues, they realized their different potentialities, one type producing pus, another cancer, and the third tubercle. . . . Why one blastema should produce pus with its abundant cells, another blastema give rise to cancer with equally abundant cells, and a third to tubercle, with very few cells, no one knows (King, 1982, p. 46).

Rudolph Virchow (1821–1902) took violent and arrogantly dogmatic exception to the blastema theory. In his opinion, tubercle developed spontaneously when cells already in the tissues degenerated, resulting in the granular substance or cheesy appearance. Writing in the 1860s, Virchow believed "that all cells arose from other pre-existing cells," a basic principle of cellular pathology that did much to eliminate blastema theory. Virchow, who did not practice medicine, was only interested in understanding cellular changes.

Jean-Antoine Villemin (1827–1892) combined his interest in the microscopic study of tissues with the clinical understanding of tuberculosis. He looked for relationships between clinical observations and pathological findings. Using his knowledge of other diseases, "Villemin was convinced that tuberculosis was a specific disease resulting from a specific infectious agent" called a "virus," which in the 1860s meant a "poison . . . that produced an effect and that had specificity." Villemin reasoned that just as other diseases like typhoid fever and plague were presumed (though not known) to be caused by a virus, so should tuberculosis be (King, 1982, pp. 55–56). Villemin argued that specific diseases could not be diagnosed only by observing the cellular evidence or any one feature. Instead, the identification of tuberculosis required correlating "granulomas in the lung with emaciation, night sweats, bronchitis, and the like" (King, 1982, p. 57). Further certainty required that he find the specific cause (virus) that produced tuberculosis. In a series of experiments Villemin was able to produce tuberculosis in rabbits by inoculating them with

caseous material and tubercles taken from various sites in man. . . . He also determined the infectious nature of sputum, bronchial secretions, and even blood. . . . Even with his limited techniques, he proved that tuberculosis was an infectious disease that could be transmitted to susceptible hosts such as the rabbit; and that a wide range of material—different types of lesions as well as sputum and (sometimes) blood—could induce the experimental disease. He also proved the "identity" of the human disease and the naturally occurring disease in cattle (King, 1982, p. 59).

This was a great step forward in the understanding of tuberculosis, establishing it as an infectious disease and sputum as an infectious agent. It happened in 1868, the year Trudeau entered medical school. This knowledge was limited to the early bacteriologists, most of whom were in Europe. Physicians were not easily convinced by experiments on animals and microscopic evidence. In 1868 it was the rare American physician who read foreign medical journals or had ever looked through a microscope.

Discovery of the infectious agent required developments in bacteriology. The prevailing thinking at the beginning of the century was that miasmata (particles) were contained in filthy air and that somehow these got into the body causing infection. One incident in Philadelphia illustrates how Benjamin Rush (1746–1813) and his colleagues thought about this noxious miasma. Assuming it had caused a severe epidemic of yellow fever, they

blamed the disease on "noxious miasma," and evil air caused by rotting matter, stagnant swamps or the breath of infected patients, [and] public minded citizens lighted fires on every street corner to burn the miasma away. A committee of doctors headed by Rush announced that fires were dangerous and probably ineffectual. When they suggested burning gunpowder instead, the citizens got their muskets down from the wall and spent the evening firing at the miasma out of the window. So many people were wounded, the mayor had to forbid this also (Coe, 1970, p. 183, quoting James T. Flexner, *Doctors on Horseback*, New York: Collier, 1962, p. 99).

In 1840, Jacob Henle, a German scientist, published *On Miasmata and Contagia*, arguing that "minute living creatures . . . parasitized the human body" causing "infectious disease" (Reiser, 1978, p. 82). In other words, the particles of miasma were not inert but were much smaller living creatures, akin to fleas and lice, which were common parasites. Building upon this idea, the French chemist Louis Pasteur (1822–1895) discovered that the decay of organic matter was associated with certain microorganisms, which were not spontaneously generated but came from the external environment. Pasteur's 1862 discovery allowed the English surgeon Joseph Lister to understand his observation that fractures where the skin was not broken healed quickly, while those that broke the skin often became infected. Realizing that the infection might be caused by bacteria in the air that infected the wound, Lister applied carbolic and phenic acid to the wounds, destroying the bacteria. As a result, infections among his surgical patients decreased impressively (Reiser, 1978, p. 83). Thanks to microscopy, by the 1860s there was strong evidence that bacteria existed and caused disease or infection. The next step for medical scientists was to discover the specific bacteria related to tuberculosis.

Robert Koch, a German physician and district health officer and a student of Jacob Henle, had attained recognition from bacteriologists for his 1877 demonstration of the causal agent in anthrax, a disease of cattle and sheep transmitted to man. After he had developed a special staining technique in his home laboratory, which enhanced the rod-shaped bacteria of tuberculosis, he was able to identify them from a variety of human and animal sources. Because these bacteria, which he called "tubercle bacilli" would not grow in the conventional media bacteriologists were using, Koch devised a new medium that nourished bacilli growth. Then he developed techniques for isolating the rod-shaped bacteria from others in order to obtain a pure culture. After growing this pure bacillus he injected it into healthy guinea pigs, reproducing the exact disease he had started with (King, 1982, p. 63). Although Villemin had established that the tuberculous material was infectious, Koch first isolated specific bacteria from that material, tubercle bacilli, which he could identify microscopically. Second, he grew the bacteria in a culture medium and, third, injected the bacteria to produce more of the same tuberculous material in healthy animals. These three steps, now known as Koch's postulates, established the tubercle bacillus as the specific cause of tuberculosis. Whenever it was present, the disease existed.

Koch announced his discovery of the tubercle bacillus in Berlin on March 24, 1882. On April 23, 1882, the *New York World* made the first report of Koch's discovery in America (Burke, 1938, p. 41).

Koch was met in the nonscientific press with a combination of indifference and skepticism. The public were most dubious about the existence of marauding germs and did not widely accept the image of a body being gobbled up by microscopic gluttons; they could not easily visualize anything doing the consuming. The most widely held belief, among doctors as well as laymen, was that the disease might be provoked by the environment, but that most fundamentally it was a manifestation of the victim's own constitution. And if that constitution chose to devour the very body in which it resided, what better proof of its dedication to the immaterial (Caldwell, 1988, pp. 21–22).

Koch's discovery did not receive serious consideration in the United States until English translations of a longer paper written in 1884 became available. After this, the disease could be accurately diagnosed by microscopic examination of autopsied lung tissue or sputum coughed up by the living patient. Discovery of the bacilli in sputum was evidence that pulmonary tuberculosis existed.

Despite the availability of these methods physicians did not routinely use them for a decade or more. An intern at Mercy Hospital in Pittsburgh wrote, "with that great disease, tuberculosis, ever about in many cases suspected to be the cause of obscure symptoms, my able chiefs never once asked for an examination for tubercle bacilli during the whole time that I was a hospital intern [1890–94], though that was already feasible" (Rosen, 1983, p. 45).

Koch's paper set off a flurry of activity lasting thirty years. This led to discoveries of tubercle bacilli in many parts of the body (e.g., nose, tonsils, eye, female breast, thymus, thyroid), the differentiation of bovine tubercle bacillus by Theobald Smith in 1896, and the culturing of the bacillus from the sickroom dust of patients (Brown, no date). Efforts were also made to kill the tubercle bacillus. Just as Joseph Lister had been able to kill the bacteria on his surgical sites, it was assumed that some antiseptic would kill the tubercle bacilli. But carbolic and phenic acid, creosote, and a variety of additional substances killed the bacilli but could not be tolerated by the animal. Nevertheless, public health physicians were able to control the bacilli by using methods of isolation and public campaigns against spitting on the streets.

The ability to identify the tubercle bacillus gave direction and certainty to clinicians who were trying to treat tuberculosis. If they could somehow eliminate the bacilli from a patient's sputum, evidence that their treatment was effective would exist. All of this was happening as Trudeau studied medicine and began to treat tuberculosis.

5

Trudeau's Reading

The reading that Trudeau began after his health improved in 1879 provided valuable information for his new sanatorium experiment.[1] One of the journals he read was the *Medical Record,* edited and published weekly by George M. Shrady, A.M., M.D., surgeon to Presbyterian and St. Francis hospitals in New York, consulting surgeon to the Hospital for Ruptured and Crippled, and president of the New York Pathological Society in 1883. The *Medical Record* contained several sections, beginning with "Editorials," in which Shrady discussed scientific controversies as well as political issues relevant to the medical profession. Often he summarized the literature on both sides of a controversy and urged his readers to settle the question by careful research. A section titled "Original Lectures" contained papers delivered at various hospitals and medical schools around the country by American and European scientists and clinicians. "Reports of Hospitals" usually contained an interesting case or two as well as the report of a treatment used on the service of a physician. "Progress of Medical Science" was a section in which Shrady reported what he judged to be important contributions to the field from French, German, Italian, Australian, English, and American medical publications. Doubtful contributions and humorous and entertaining medical claims were usually relegated to a section labeled "Medical Items and News." "Reports of Societies" covered local, state, national, and international society meetings. "Original Communications" included papers solicited from and submitted by leading authorities. Finally, there were sections for "Correspondence" and "Reviews and Notices of Books." The *Medical Record* contained the current thinking from the "science" of medicine as seen through the eyes of an orthodox physician from the New York City establishment who agreed to the "Code of Ethics" adopted by the American Medical Association (*Medical Record*, vol. 1, March 1, 1866, p. 14).

Another journal mentioned by Trudeau is the *American Journal of Medical Science,* edited by Isaac Hays, A.M., M.D. This was an older journal in its seventy-seventh volume by 1879. In the 1880s there appear to have been very few articles stressing bacteriology and experimental medicine and more articles expressing clinical opinions of practitioners about how to treat patients based on their experience.

A third journal, *Medical News and Abstracts*, was in its thirty-seventh volume by 1879. It summarized publications from Europe and the United States. It appears to be quite similar to the *Medical Record*, summarizing research on phthisis and presenting a variety of treatments as they were published.

While these journals contained most of what was available, the popular press regularly published scientific news about consumption, the major cause of death much feared by the public. As journal publishing was a source of income for the editor, there tended to be considerable overlap, especially in reporting information taken from various foreign journals like *Lancet*.

In this mix of information it is difficult to know what impressed Trudeau.[2] However, it is likely that he tested the articles he read against his own experience as a tuberculosis patient and the experiences of those he had already treated prior to 1884.

Trudeau said he began reading these journals in 1879, eleven years after beginning medical school. Although he had been taught that phthisis was "a non-contagious, generally incurable and inherited disease," medical science was rapidly changing. Trudeau must have discovered this as he perused his journals. There were at least two important and unsolved questions with respect to tuberculosis, which was then called "phthisis" by those who spoke the medical dialect and called "consumption" by journalists and the masses. First was the question of etiology, or cause. Was phthisis inherited or contagious? If inherited, one could do little to prevent it. If contagious, then the physician had a role in prevention or intervening in the causal process. Second was the question of prognosis. Was death inevitable, or could people survive the disease? If survival was possible, then the physician had a greater role in caring for the patient to encourage survival. Instead of just making the dying patient comfortable, he could aggressively treat the disease and restore the patient to health. The journals in 1877–78 contain many references to these issues and allow us a picture of Trudeau's field just before he began reading in 1879.

ETIOLOGY

The idea that phthisis was inherited had been challenged in France in 1868 by the bacteriologist Villemin, who had established that it was an infectious disease and sputum was the infectious agent. But American clinical practitioners had a long way to go before these scientific ideas were widely accepted. When Henry I. Bowditch, a physician and public health advocate from Massachusetts, surveyed 210 physicians on the "Causes and Antecedents of Consumption" in the early 1870s, 205 said that the disease was caused or promoted by hereditary influences (Teller, 1988, p. 8).

Conflicting American ideas about etiology are illustrated by comments such as that of Dr. Gleitsmann of Baltimore, who stated that "the percentage of [phthisis] deaths in the spring months is shown to be larger than in the other seasons, and this is accounted for by the humidity of the atmosphere and the frequent thaws and rains" (*Medical Record*, vol. 12, 1877, p. 370). At the twenty-eighth annual meeting (1877) of the American Medical Association (AMA) in Chicago, Dr. A. N. Bell of Brooklyn "spoke at length of the danger of imbibing tubercular consumption through milch cows, by the use of milk from the cows infected with the disease. The fact that tuberculosis was transmissible was an undoubted one" (*Medical Record*, vol. 12, 1877, p. 389). However, at the next AMA annual meeting much debate over climate achieved little agreement in the report of the section on Practical Medicine, June 4, 1878.

Dr. F. H. Davis of Chicago, read a paper . . . in which he maintained that the influence of climate in the production of tuberculosis was overrated. More powerful causes were want of exercise, improper clothing of the body, and dampness. Dr. Dennison of Colorado, spoke of moisture as an element in the production of phthisis, especially moisture such as the inmates were exposed to in houses which were built upon soil more or less filled with water, as in many cities. Dr. Lester of Kansas City . . . did not believe that moisture had any special influence in the development of phthisis, and cited as evidence the fact that in many localities consumption was unknown while the forests remained undisturbed, but as soon as they were cleared off phthisis appeared (*Medical Record*, vol. 13, June 29, 1878, p. 504).

Environmental factors were considered important, also,

A change from agricultural to manufacturing pursuits was regarded as an important factor in the production of phthisis. As illustrative of that view reference was made to Swedish and Norwegian immigrants, who usually came from agricultural districts, but when they arrived in this country many of them engaged in manufacturing pursuits, their children as domestics, and among them phthisis was of frequent occurrence (*Medical Record*, vol. 13, June 29, 1878, p. 504).

While the AMA clinicians were arguing among themselves using clinical experience for evidence, the editor Shrady seemed convinced that phthisis was contagious and reported from the *Hospital Gazette* that

Dr. Tappeiner has proved by experiments in Buhl's laboratory at Monaco, that phthisis is contagious. He mixed the sputa of consumptives with water, and made five dogs inhale the mixture in the form of spray. Two dogs were also made to swallow a portion. After a lapse of six weeks the dogs were killed. They presented a general miliary tuberculosis of lungs, liver, and kidneys, and, in the two who had swallowed the matter, of the digestive apparatus, also. Carmine, which had been mixed with the inhaled liquid, was found in the pulmonary cells. It is suggested that these experiments are an indication that the air of badly ventilated apartments occupied by phthisical patients may become dangerous to healthy persons (*Medical Record,* vol. 14, October 19, 1878, p. 313).

In June 1877, Professor Klebs announced in Munich that "tuberculosis was an infectious disease of parasitic nature . . . introduced by certain micro-organisms which invaded the body and multiplied in it." He held out the hope that curing tuberculosis could occur if these organisms could be annihilated (*Medical News and Abstracts*, vol. 38, April 1880, pp. 276–331, from the *British Medical Journal*, January 1880).

Clinical accounts like the following argued against heredity and for contagion. In the *London Medical Record* for July 15, 1880, a Norwegian physician described cases in which

a phthisical man married a healthy woman. He died, she became phthisical as well as her sister who lived with them. The sister married a healthy man who became phthisical as well as his sister's daughter who lived with them. One of their children died of meningitis and two showed signs of pulmonary tubercle. The girl who served the first man's wife became tuberculous and died (*Medical News and Abstracts*, vol. 38, September 1880, pp. 532–33).

From these brief quotations several conclusions can be drawn. Trudeau's teacher Alonzo Clark's idea that phthisis was "non-contagious and inherited" was no longer popular. While clinicians argued about the effects of climate, they at least acknowledged that certain conditions were more likely to produce disease and that certain substances, sputum or milk from cows with bovine tuberculosis, might be a source of the contagion. Despite the adequacy of their arguments, usually from clinical experience or opinion unsubstantiated by facts, they acknowledged phthisis to be contagious. Bacteriologists, especially those in Europe, were convinced that phthisis was contagious and were actively searching for the specific germ that conveyed the disease to humans. Having successfully fought a cholera epidemic, preventing its introduction to New York City in 1865–66 by public hygiene methods (which assumed contagion as a principle), some American physicians were primed to think of other diseases in a similar way. Whatever the cause, it was possible to think of tuberculosis contagion as a parasitic mechanism. When Trudeau returned to the medical literature in 1879, his original assumptions about tuberculosis were being challenged.

PROGNOSIS

Although Trudeau had been taught that tuberculosis was generally incurable, it was obvious that he had survived and returned to a fairly adequate level of functioning. He had experienced Alonzo Clark's general treatment while recuperating at Paul Smith's. That there was hope for people with the disease must have been part of his own thinking, despite his brother's experience.

At the 1877 AMA meeting in Chicago there was general agreement that phthisis could and should be treated. At least in the early stages, change of climate was considered beneficial and high altitudes, like Colorado, attractive (*Medical Record*, vol. 12, June 16, 1877, p. 378–79). Dr. Francis Delafield, adjunct professor of pathology and practical medicine, published a clinical lecture given at the College of Physicians and Surgeons in which he presented the case of a forty-two-year-old man who originally spat blood in 1864, improved until it happened again in 1869, and then returned to work until March 1876, when he again raised blood, lost flesh, and was too weak to work. Despite this history, Delafield claimed his "prognosis is tolerably good. If the man takes proper care of himself he may live for a long time. The treatment is entirely constitutional. He might be benefited perhaps by a change of climate, and he should take tonics and cod-liver oil. No local treatment whatever is required" (*Medical Record*, vol. 12, May 12, 1877, p. 306).

Similar positive results were suggested by Dr. McCall Anderson, of Glasgow, in an article excerpted from the *Lancet* of March 24 and 31, 1877. Three cases of acute phthisis that recovered under his care are described:

The treatment consisted in iced cloths to the abdomen for half an hour every two hours, and in the internal administration of quinine . . . digitalis . . . and opium . . . with the view of reducing the fever . . . used wither alone or conjointly. . . .

The profuse sweats were checked by hypodermic injections of atrophine . . . at night. . . .

The bowels were kept open by enemata or by oil. . . . In order to keep up the strength of the patients, milk and soups, with brandy or champagne were administered in small quantities at frequent intervals. In one case carbonate of ammonia was given (*Medical Record*, vol. 12, May 5, 1877, p. 296).

Dr. Anderson spoke often "On the Curability of Attacks of Acute Phthisis," making similar statements to the British Medical Association in 1880 (*Medical News and Abstracts*, vol. 38, October 1880, p. 611). Shrady wrote,

The treatment of localized cavities in the lung by injections of dilute Lugol's solution [Lugol's caustic solution, consisting of one part each of iodine and potassium iodide dissolved in two parts of water], originally introduced by Professor Pepper, has been discussed in the medical press. Further experience with it has confirmed the belief that it is most valuable in some cases as favoring the contraction and cicatrization [healing which leaves a scar] of cavities. It is in no case attended with any dangerous consequences. . . .

More recently Lugol's solution has been injected into lung-tissue in cases of incipient phthisis. In one case, recently discharged from the hospital, the treatment was pursued nearly every week for a number of months. The disease was arrested, the physical signs disappeared, the general symptoms greatly improved, and the patient was discharged apparently well!

Dr. Pepper says his method deserves further study (*Medical Record*, vol. 12, p. 182).

Other cures are reported to use ergot as a fluid extract and in pill form (*Medical Record*, vol. 12, November 3, 1877, pp. 707–10), tincture of silphium (*Medical Record*, vol. 14, September 7, 1878, p. 198), inhalations of carbolic acid, cod-liver oil, iodide of potassium, and a liberal diet (*Medical Record*, vol. 13, April 20, 1878, pp. 330–32). "Dr. Pocagnik, of Vienna, is a warm advocate for cold sponging in phthisis" (*Medical Record*, vol. 13, June 1, 1878, p. 440. The humor is the editor's). Discussion of a variety of treatments implied that phthisis was treatable. While there was no agreement about a specific method of treatment, there was some agreement about the goals of treatment: Deterioration of the lungs should be stopped. Consumption of the body should be reversed and weight, energy, and well-being restored, usually by rest and diet. After these two goals were achieved the disease might be arrested.

When Trudeau returned to the medical literature in 1879, it was fortunate that he was advised to read these journals, which covered the sciences relevant to medicine as well as the art of clinical practice. Bacteriology was beginning to make important scientific contributions that revolutionized medical practice, and the editor of the *Medical Record*, George Shrady, was well aware of this.

The period between Trudeau's medical school and his return to reading the medical journals is described by John Warner.

Between the mid-1860s and the mid-1880s, some American physicians began to articulate an expansive program for reconstructing medicine on the foundation of experimental science. The claim of laboratory science to practical relevance in medical therapeutics did much more than challenge the reign of empiricism: it urged a thorough going rearrangement of the relationships among therapeutic practice, knowledge, and professional identity. As the proponents of the newly laid basis for treatment teased out the implications of physiological therapeutics, they portrayed it as an integral part of a new medical ethos gradually taking shape (Warner, 1986, p. 258).

Perhaps it was this shift in medicine that led Trudeau to subscribe to medical journals in the first place. If he hoped to establish a reputation while isolated in the deep Adirondack woods, not many options existed. Local people were impressed by this dignified but frail gentleman who raised money to establish Episcopal churches and cared for anyone regardless of the fee. It is likely that his fluency in

French appealed to many of the local French Canadian woodsmen who had moved to the area to cut the forests. And his slightly accented English gave an aura of continental sophistication, that undoubtedly impressed many of the wealthy summer visitors and camp owners. The hunting and fishing guides who were the major source of tourist revenues welcomed an enterprise that would attract business to the area and contributed land to develop the sanitarium. Summer visitors whom Trudeau treated were charged low fees and urged to contribute to whatever charity the doctor was raising money for at the time.

Among these summer vacationers were physicians like Alfred Loomis. He had witnessed Trudeau's recovery from a very poor prognosis over the years and wrote an article describing his case as well as other cases including his own. The article did much to publicize the Adirondack area among eastern physicians, and Loomis agreed to refer patients to Trudeau's experiment in sanitarium care (*Medical Record*, vol. 15, April 26 and May 3, 1879, pp. 385–89 and 409–12). But the chief claim to prominence and recognition was a connection to laboratory and experimental science. Though Trudeau's clinical and gentlemanly social skills could impress his patients, his reputation in the new world of medicine depended upon his knowledge as a scientist. To that end, reading the medical literature was a beginning step.

In 1879, as Trudeau began studying, younger medical graduates no longer believed what he had been taught about tuberculosis. Medicine was benefiting from experimental laboratory science. In fifty years, the number of medical journals had increased from eight in the United States to "fifty-three of the regular school, nine homeopathic, and seven eclectic" (*Medical Record,* vol. 15, February 8, 1879, p. 143).

The universities were training chemists, physicists, biologists, geologists, astronomers, and mathematicians. By 1880, "the American scientific community included some 3300 practitioners, people who to some degree used science in their employment. . . . Affiliated with the practitioners was a group of cultivators . . . aficionados, friends and gadabouts of science, men and women who attended public scientific lectures and read *Popular Science Monthly*" (Kevles, Sturchio, and Carroll, 1980, p. 27). These scientists were supported by wealthy sponsors. "The religious impulse had often combined with the desire for social prestige to point the way for new wealth to gain respectability by endowing good scientific works. Thus, both philanthropy and public subscription had fostered the establishment of numerous astronomical observatories in the United States, an estimated 144 of them by 1882, probably more than in any other nation" (Kevles, Sturchio, and Carroll, 1980, p. 30). If science were to save the world, the wealthy wanted to be connected with it. Besides a genuine interest in medicine and the desire to support his family, a similar impulse may have motivated Trudeau to read the medical literature in 1879. Thinking of his sanatorium as a "scientific experiment" certainly tapped into the general enthusiasm.

1879–1884: TRUDEAU READS MEDICAL JOURNALS

From 1879, when Trudeau began his reeducation, until the summer of 1884, when he decided to begin his experiment in sanitorium care, the medical literature covered a variety of topics reflecting the general changes occurring in medical science and the medical profession. The developing methods of science were influencing work in the laboratory, but empirical methods dominated in clinical practice. Acceptable clinical arguments could be made using associations and correlations backed up by the physician's personal stature and testimony. Phthisis deaths could be associated with spring thaws and rains, cleared forests, and manufacturing. And these factors were argued to be causal with confidence and conviction because physicians had experienced them.

At the same time the germ theory of disease received considerable publicity. The question was no longer whether there were germs; rather, it was how best to prevent them from infecting a surgical site. Joseph Lister had visited the United States in 1876 to describe his surgical techniques; and George Shrady, also a surgeon, commented,

The theory on which Mr. Lister insists as the cause of putrefaction, non-union, and its attendant results, is that known as the germ theory, and to prevent these germs from planting themselves in the wound is the aim of all antiseptic precaution.

Mr. Lister and those who have followed closely in his footsteps, have certainly obtained better results than those who have treated wounds on the old plan. But other surgeons who have treated their amputations in accordance with plans diametrically opposed to the antiseptic method as proposed by Mr. Lister, or who have omitted certain precautions which Mr. Lister has insisted upon as being essential, have had as good results as claimed by those who followed strict antiseptic rules as laid down by him. We think it is time to examine this question of the treatment of wounds, and see if a careful review of the different methods will not point out what are essential and what may be discarded.

Shrady then analyzed five different methods of treating amputations and after what would now be called a meta-analysis summarized that all of them insist on

perfect drainage, cleanliness, and rest. The plan of Mr. Lister is expensive, requires considerable experience, and more personal supervision than any of the other methods and at the same time more handling of the parts; and the question arises. Is it superior to any of the others, and cannot equally good results be obtained by a modification? . . . There is growing conviction that the spray [Lister's spray] can be dispensed with, and that a thorough washing of the cut surfaces with an antiseptic fluid will accomplish the same end. . . . If we were called upon to decide what was the most important element in Mr. Lister's dressing, we should say that it was his system of drainage, and to this more than anything else must be attributed his success (*Medical Record,* vol. 15, March 1, 1879, pp. 206–8).

A comment published three weeks later by Faneuil D. Weise, Professor of Practical and Surgical Anatomy in the Medical Department of the University of the City of New York, argued that the key to the five methods discussed is "cleanliness." "The prevention of germ implantation from the air, upon the surface of the wound . . . to the carrying out of this latter indication must be credited the wonderful successes of antiseptic surgery. . . . Antiseptic surgery, by preventing putrefaction [decomposition] in the wound, has given a precision to surgical prognosis . . . it has broadened the field of operative surgery, which without its protective influence would be unwarranted" (*Medical Record,* vol. 15, March 22, 1879, pp. 269–70). Weise believed that germs were important, and Shrady acknowledged their importance by using his editorial judgement to print this comment.

In the June 14, 1879, issue, Shrady reported a paper by Dr. Perrin from the Union Medicale that advocated alcohol spray in the place of Lister's carbolic acid.

Mr. Perrin claims that he has made a number of experiments, which seem to prove that carbolic spray has really no influence on the evolution of atmospheric germs in liquids suitable for their culture, and on the consequent phenomena of putrefaction. On the other hand, alcohol diluted with an equal volume of water, he says, acts on the soil, that is, the wound; renders albuminous liquid imputresible; has considerable coagulating power, readily stops bleeding from vessels of small caliber, quickly moistens cotton; and penetrates the tissues of the body, without having the instant action of carbolic acid. . . .

Mr. Perrin now positively asserts that he has demonstrated by experiments that the carbolic acid spray has no influence on the evolution of atmospheric germs in liquids suitable for their culture. The issue being clearly stated, let this point satisfactorily be settled, and as it is capable of practical demonstration by simple tests we trust it will be done at once. This is a matter of great importance to the medical profession, and highly interesting in its scientific bearings. We know many whose decision on this question would be received with respect and we confidently look to them for a prompt solution (*Medical Record,* vol. 15, June 14, 1879, p. 561).

As a surgeon interested in establishing the medical profession on the foundation of laboratory science, he encouraged a test of Lister's methods by publishing relevant and often conflicting points of view.

In this context of increasing popularity for the germ theory, the contagiousness of tuberculosis became a prominent question. On February 7, 1880, Shrady reported in the "Progress of Medical Science" section: "Professor Cohnheim declares himself in favor of the view that all tubercular processes are infective in origin. Dr. Schueppel thinks that bacteria underlie them, and hence the appropriateness of all anti-parasitic remedies" (*Medical Record,* vol. 17, February 7, 1880, p. 147). On June 26, 1880, in the same section Shrady reported,

Referring to Prof. Cohnheim's latest views on the contagiousness of tuberculosis, Dr. Freidlander remarks: The power of communicating contagion is an indisputable property of all tubercular affections. . . . (the) characteristic infection occurred without exception in every instance where tubercular substance was employed for inoculation. . . .

The carriers of infection are presumably parasitic organisms. Tubercular virus commonly enters the system by inhalation through the respiratory passages. Thus the primary lesion is frequently found in the lungs whence the disease may be carried to the pleura and the bronchial glands, or, through the agency of the sputa to the alimentary canal. This produces the common form of pneumo-intestinal phthisis. The intestinal tract is also liable to direct infection through the agency of diseased cow's milk (*Medical Record,* vol. 17, June 26, 1880, pp. 723–24).

In July 1880 Shrady published an original communication, "The Contagion of Consumption," by James T. Whittaker, M.D., Professor of the Theory and Practice of Medicine, Medical College of Ohio. Whittaker tried to explain why the profession resisted the idea that tuberculosis was contagious.

What has especially prevented the general acceptance of the infectiousness of tuberculosis is the widespread belief in the almost exclusively hereditary transmission of the disease. . . . Because members of the same family succumb to the disease, is not so much proof of the influence of heredity as of contagion, for a like implication is seen in all kinds of infectious disease among individuals in close association. And it is the observation of every practitioner of experience, that a large contingent of cases develop entirely independent of heredity. . . .

The whole question of the contagion of consumption, i.e., of the specificity of the tuberculous virus, hinges upon its inoculability, and of this capability there is now scarcely room for doubt.

Following Cohnheim, Whittaker argued that tuberculosis was very similar to syphilis.

Syphilis . . . reaches the body through organs of generation, while tuberculosis is breathed, for the most part, into the lungs, or is swallowed with food, as with milk, the most frequent cause of tuberculosis in childhood. . . .

It is also true of both diseases that they are in the vast majority of cases not inherited, but acquired. . . . Bad air, food, or drink are productive of tuberculosis only when they contain the virus of the disease (*Medical Record,* vol. 18, July 24, 1880, pp. 90–93).

Despite this strong argument for the contagiousness of tuberculosis, Shrady wrote an editorial, "Study Phthisis," stating

These are troublous times for the student who wishes to gain clear pathological ideas on the subject of phthisis. If educated a decade ago he was probably first brought to believe the views of Virchow and Niemeyer, that chronic phthisis is a scrofulous inflammation of the lung, with which tubercles might or might not be

associated. . . . Then he learned there were at least three types of phthisis (Ruehle)
. . . that it begins generally with bronchitis (Rindfleisch). . . . results from a specific
infection, the tubercular virus; that phthisis is analogous to syphilis.

Avoiding the question of the contagiousness of tuberculosis Shrady commented on treatment: "We advise the student to stick to his Neimeyer and give
cod-liver oil, while waiting for the better settlement of the pathology and
classification of phthisis" (*Medical Record,* vol. 18, July 24, 1880, p. 98).

But the question of the infectious nature of tuberculous materials persisted. Shrady summarized the work of a French scientist: "M. Martin then
sought to determine whether or not the tubercles produced by the inoculation
of tubercular matter differed in other respects from those following ordinary
inoculations. He found that the tubercles of tuberculosis possessed the
property of infection, whereas the pseudo-tubercle lacked this quality" (*Gaz.
med. de Paris*, January 22, 1881; *Medical Record,* vol. 19, March 5, 1881).
Shrady concluded two weeks later, saying, "Now it seems to have been
demonstrated that tuberculosis can be transmitted from man to the lower
animals and from one of the lower animals to another. The only point about
which there is doubt is whether tuberculosis can be conveyed from the lower
animals to man through their flesh or milk" (*Medical Record,* vol. 19, March
19, 1881, p. 323). Bovine tuberculosis was common in cattle and had long
been suspected of causing human tuberculosis. From an article in the *Journal
of Comparative Medicine* Shrady suggested a way to study this problem:

There is . . . only one certain way by which the question whether man can be infected by
the milk or flesh of tuberculous cattle can be settled. This is by making the experiment upon
man himself—upon criminals condemned to death. There is nothing cruel or at all revolting
to the idea. For a certain period previous to the day for execution, the person to be
experimented on should be fed with the milk or flesh, or both, of tuberculous cattle. . . . The
criminal's condition should be carefully watched to see whether tubercles develop. After
execution a careful necropsy should be held. By experiments conducted in this way, results
of the highest importance to science and preventive medicine could be secured (*Medical
Record,* vol. 19, March 19, 1991, p. 323).

This research on human subjects was acceptable in the 1880s, and in 1882
Shrady reported an actual experiment from Greece under "Medical Items and
News":

Two Greek physicians have recently made a direct experiment to see whether
bovine tuberculosis could be inoculated in man. The subject of the experiment was
a common laborer, who in consequence of arterial occlusion, was slowly perishing
from progressive gangrene of the leg. In other respects the patient was healthy, and
a careful examination showed that the lungs were in normal condition. As he refused
to submit to the amputation of the limb, pronounced necessary to save his life, his

medical attendants decided to test by direct experiment whether tubercle can be propagated from phthisical cows to man by inoculation. A quantity of tuberculous matter was accordingly injected into the circulation, whether with or without consent is not specified. The man lived about six weeks, then died of blood poisoning inseparable from progressive gangrene. The autopsy disclosed the existence of well-defined tuberculous deposits, without abscess or other disease of the pulmonary organ, very small, evidently very recent, and as the daring experimentalists argued, the direct result of the inoculation (*Medical Record,* vol. 22, September 9, 1882, pp. 307–8).

Shrady collected further evidence for comparing bovine and human tuberculosis from the *Dublin Journal of Medical Science*, May 1881. Under "Progress of Medical Science" he wrote:

Dr. Creighton contends that there is strong evidence from the anatomical similarity between the disease in the cow and that often observed in man, that the infection is very commonly communicated to the human subject by the milk of cows affected with perlsucht, or as he calls it, bovine tuberculosis. . . .

Milk is now recognized as a means of carrying the virus of disease. . . .

Dr. Creighton states the view that many of these supposed attacks of typhoid fever are in reality outbreaks of tuberculosis, and that the milk was contaminated, not by adulteration, but owing to its having been secreted by tuberculous cows (*Medical Record,* vol. 19, June 18, 1881, p. 685).

One would have thought that physicians would be able to accept the evidence that tuberculous materials injected into animals produced evidence of tuberculosis in the animals like tubercles in the lungs. However, they began to inject other foreign substances under the skin and discovered they could produce tuberculosis with these substances, also (*Medical Record,* vol. 21, March 4, 1882, p. 234).

This controversy was finally put to rest for the *Medical Record,* when William T. Belfield's lecture "On the Relations of Micro-organisms to Disease" was published in the Original Lectures section. Belfield, lecturer on pathology and on the genito-urinary diseases at Rush Medical College, in Chicago, was giving the Cartwright Lectures to the Alumni Association of the College of Physicians and Surgeons. It is not known whether Trudeau attended the meeting but it is likely that he read these lectures, as they were given at his alma mater.

In 1865 Villemin demonstrated that the subcutaneous introduction of tuberculous human tissue was followed by local and general tuberculosis in rabbits and guinea pigs. His results were in succeeding years corroborated by Klebs, Lebert, Waldenburg, Cohnheim, Frankel, Tappeiner, Orth, Bolinger—in short by all who made the experiment. . . . Tuberculosis can, therefore, according to the unanimous testimony of observers, be induced by inoculation with tuberculous tissue. But it soon became doubtful whether this unquestioned fact could be interpreted as proof that there is anything specific about the tubercle; for it is evident that if all the effects produced by inoculation with tubercle can be just as certainly induced by non-tuberculous material, no assumption of specific nature is necessary. It was demonstrated by Burden-Sanderson, Wilson, Fox, Martin, Waldenberg, Cohnheim, Frankel . . . after the induction of irritation and inflammation in the subcutaneous tissue or peritoneum, an eruption of miliary tubercles, indistinguishable histologically from those following inoculations with tuberculous matter, often occurred. . . .

Klebs suggested that the successful induction of tuberculosis after the insertion of glass, wood, etc., might after all be simply infection from contact with animals already tuberculous, or from tuberculous materials left in laboratories by previous subjects of the disease.

Recognizing this possibility of contamination, Cohnheim and Frankel repeated their experiments using isolated animals and presumably sterilizing the injected materials, and none of their animals had any evidence of tuberculosis.

Belfield, applauding the role of scientists, concluded, "Cohnheim, with the moral courage born of true scientific spirit, published this fact, and acknowledged the justice of Kleb's suggestion" (*Medical Record,* vol. 23, March 10, 1883, pp. 253–57).

By 1883 the contagiousness of tuberculosis seemed to be fairly well accepted by laboratory scientists. But this required that the reality of germs and their ability to contaminate animals and laboratory materials be recognized. Kleb's suggestion that experimental animals and injected materials could have been contaminated by the tuberculosis bacillus was an important step in acceptance of the germ theory.

While the evidence from laboratory researchers convinced scientists like Belfield, he admitted that there were still

many practicing physicians who cannot believe that tuberculosis is communicable . . . because clinical proof to that effect is unsatisfactory . . . a surgeon pricks his finger in dressing a pyaemic patient, and in twenty-four hours has a chill and local symptoms pointing unmistakably to the source of infection . . . an observer . . . might honestly believe that the infection which manifests itself weeks or months later is spontaneous . . . because they see no striking symptoms to mark the hour or the day of infection, insist that no infection has occurred.

The opportunities for the usual mode of infection by syphilis are only occasional; and the attendant circumstances are such to impress such occasions upon the mind and conscience; when therefore, the first evidence of infection appears, perhaps weeks subsequently, upon that part of the anatomy peculiarly exposed upon such an occasion, it is but normal that the mind should associate the two phenomena as cause and effect. Were syphilis communicated not in the way at present in vogue but by inhalation; were the initial evidence of infection not upon the integuments and therefore visible, but in the lungs and hence inaccessible to the eye, there might be the same clinical grounds for doubting the infectiousness of syphilis as of tuberculosis (*Medical Record,* vol. 23, March 10, 1882, p. 256).

Tuberculosis had been discovered to have a twenty- to thirty-day incubation period, and this clinical analogy with syphilis illustrated that point very well for the male clinicians in Belfield's audience. In the 1980s physicians and the public have had to overcome similar shortcomings in their thinking to accommodate the idea that the AIDS virus may have a seven- to ten-year incubation period.

The evidence that had convinced Belfield and many other American laboratory scientists had been presented a year earlier by Robert Koch in Berlin. It had been widely publicized in the scientific and popular literature. Shrady's editorial of May 20, 1882, recognized "Koch's Discovery of Tubercular Parasite":

A paper recently read by Dr. Robert Koch before the Berlin Physiological Society has attracted wide attention. Dr. Koch here makes some very positive announcements regarding the etiology of tuberculosis. Whether his views and conclusions be right or not, the facts that he relates are novel and interesting. . . .

Koch claims a positive universality for these organisms in all tuberculous tissues. It is, he thinks, the organized virus of tuberculosis which Cohnheim and others have despaired of finding. . . .

Koch states that in the sputa of the phthisical the bacilli are always found.

After describing Koch's methodology, Shrady stated,

Dr. Koch believes that tuberculosis is a contagious disease, and that the sputa and exhalations of the phthisical are dangerous. He also believes the milk and flesh of tuberculous cows to be a source of danger. . . . We confess to some scepticism regarding the facts, and still more to their far reaching significance. . . . The practical conclusions that we must especially guard against the disease by disinfecting the sputa and breath of the phthisical, and by avoiding the disease or its products in lower animals, are so at variance with what most previous experience has taught that the profession will demand much further explanation and confirmation before such views are accepted (*Medical Record,* vol. 21, May 20, 1882, pp. 547–48).

These cautious and reluctant comments by Shrady in 1882 were to be contradicted when he published Belfield's lecture the next year.

While in 1882 the laboratory scientists rushed to replicate Koch's work, the clinicians were as skeptical as Shrady. William H. Welch, who had studied in Europe, "demonstrated the discovery before his laboratory class at Bellevue"; but Alfred Loomis, Trudeau's mentor, a respected clinician and diagnostician, "gave his judgement by peering about him and saying to applause, 'People say there are bacteria in the air, but I cannot see them.' To this Welch, who would later develop the new medical school at Johns Hopkins, commented: 'That's too bad. Loomis is such a nice man' " (Fleming, 1954, p. 72). Much later Loomis wrote Trudeau he would approve of the new edition of the *Practice of*

Medicine, in which Loomis finally accepted the reality of germs (Trudeau, 1915, p. 175).

Trudeau said he read an abstract of Koch's discovery in a medical journal in 1883. Whether this was Shrady's editorial of May 20, 1882, which was an abstract from the German, or whether it was Belfield's Cartwright lectures published March 10, 1883, we cannot be sure, as Belfield also summarized Koch's work. If Trudeau's date is accurate, perhaps it is the Belfield lecture he is referring to. In any case, Trudeau, if he wasn't by now convinced of the contagiousness of tuberculosis from his own personal experience, was so impressed by Koch's discovery that he wanted to reproduce Koch's work for himself. Unable to read German, Trudeau complained about this to his friend C. M. Lea, the Philadelphia medical publisher and husband of an early private summer patient, and received a translation as a gift at Christmas that year (Trudeau, 1901). Impressed by Koch's paper, Trudeau wanted to learn bacteriology immediately. Though he had a microscope he did not know the proper staining techniques for revealing the bacillus and knew nothing about growing the bacillus as a culture. On his next trip to New York City Trudeau prevailed upon Dr. T. Mitchell Prudden, who had been recently employed by the College of Physicians and Surgeons to teach in a new subject area for American medical schools, namely, pathology. Prudden had worked in Koch's laboratory and, along with his assistant Dr. Hodenpyl, taught Trudeau the bacteriology necessary to replicate Koch's experiments. (Prudden, like Trudeau's father, had a strong interest in American Indians and carried out studies of the Anasazi remains in the Southwest.) Once Trudeau had perfected this laboratory technique he examined the sputum of all patients to be certain they carried the bacilli and thus had tuberculosis. After succeeding in the replication of Koch's experiments, he obtained the tubercle bacillus in pure culture. This led to a series of events that convinced not only him but many of his clinical colleagues of the significance of Koch's work. By the mid-1880s, Trudeau believed that germs did exist and that a specific germ, the tubercle bacillus, was the cause of the contagious disease, tuberculosis.

But there was another issue that bothered many clinicians, especially those who believed that heredity and a person's constitution were important.

THE SELF-LIMITING NATURE OF TUBERCULOSIS

If tuberculosis were a contagious and fatal disease how was it possible that some people who had the disease did not die, but recovered? Clinicians who worked with tuberculosis patients noted that very few nurses and hospital personnel contracted the disease (*Medical Record,* vol. 22, no. 14. September 30, 1882, p. 388). Shrady noted that "Dr. Heitler, of Vienna, found in 16,562 autopsies, 780 cases of 'absolute tubercular patches.' Of these 503 were in men, 277 in women. It is inferred that they represent cases in which the phthisical process spontaneously ceased" (*Medical Record,* vol. 18, October 9, 1880, p. 392).

In a paper, "Self Limitation in Cases of Phthisis," presented at the New York Academy of Medicine, May 15, 1879, Dr. Austin Flint suggested that "there were certain cases which exemplified a tendency to recovery." In other words, the disease was "self-limiting." Dr. Flint often cited a famous essay by Jacob Bigelow of Boston on the self-limiting character of certain diseases, and it is this idea that he adopted (Flint, 1874, p. 19, 128). Referring to cases already published in his book on phthisis, he said it was difficult to decide whether the treatment had been the cure or whether the cure had been spontaneous. If people could recover spontaneously from tuberculosis, then what was the role of the physician? The discussion of Flint's paper concluded that humans had a "tendency to spontaneous recovery" and the physician's role was "to assist nature." Changes in climate would remove the person from the irritating agent and good nutrition would assist the body in fighting the disease (*Medical Record,* vol. 16, July 19, 1879, pp. 65–66).

No longer was a person's genetic or constitutional background an explanation for getting the disease; rather, one's general health and general working and living conditions were important. One month earlier at the New York Academy of Medicine, Dr. James R. Leaming had said that tuberculosis always had a "predisposing cause in some depression of the vital force which might be due to various circumstances. Thus any individual who had long been attendant upon the sick, the student unsuccessful in passing his examination, the man of business perplexed with unusual care, the disappointed lover, the defeated soldier were all peculiarly liable to be attacked" (*Medical Record,* vol. 15, May 3, 1879, p. 427). A "change of climate" could therefore mean many things: removal from irritating and noxious air at work or at home, avoiding a stressful social situation, and experiencing a new set of scenic and climatic conditions. This is essentially what Alonzo Clark had taught about climate to medical students at the College of Physicians and Surgeons. In order to rebuild the body, "to assist nature," a "change of climate," especially in the early stages of the disease, was a popular treatment. Certainly Trudeau must have felt very comfortable with this idea, as that is what he had done. But the "climates" of Aiken, South Carolina, and St. Paul, Minnesota, had not helped him, whereas resting in the Adirondacks had reduced his fever and restored his health. His "passion for the wild out-of-door existence" made this particular change of climate favorable for his "restoration to health."

CLIMATE AS A TREATMENT FOR TUBERCULOSIS

As we have seen, "change of climate" came to mean many things. Trudeau's professor, Alonzo Clark, had suggested going to the mountains and becoming a stage driver. He encouraged people with early tuberculosis to get away from the cold winds and the poverty and filth of cities. A survey of New York City in 1865 "showed that conditions in that city were as bad as those anywhere in the civilized world and that the existing city agencies were far too corrupt and inefficient to correct them" (Teller, 1988, p. 13).

Now that tuberculosis was far more amenable to treatment than earlier thought, one of the fashionable treatments became that which wealthy people had been able to use for a long time—a change of climate by escaping the cities. Dr. C. Theodore Williams reported "Cases of Phthisis Treated at High Altitudes" in the *Lancet* of August 16, 1879, describing the influence of a mountain climate "as intensely stimulating . . . appetite increases, digestion and assimilation improves. . . . The effect on the lungs is chiefly the result of the rarefied air combined with exercise" (*American Journal of the Medical Sciences*, vol. 78, October 1879, p. 564).

The Adirondack climate was recommended by Trudeau's mentor, Dr. A. L. Loomis, Professor of the Theory and Practice of Medicine in the Medical Department of New York University. His paper, which had been read to the Medical Society of the State of New York, was called "The Adirondack Region as a Therapeutical Agent in the Treatment of Pulmonary Phthisis" and was published in *Medical Record,* vol. 15, April 26 and May 3, 1879. The cases presented include himself, Trudeau, and others whom Trudeau had supervised for Loomis. Admitting that the "Adirondack region may be considered a moist, cool climate" with many overcast days, he argued that the purity of the air is an important factor. When a southern trip had not relieved his symptoms Loomis spent the summer of 1867 in the Adirondacks.

My personal experience that summer convinced me that there was something in the air of this region especially adapted to diseased lungs; that, if the climate had no direct influence in arresting or preventing phthisical developments, it certainly allayed bronchial irritation, and the phthisical invalid soon became able to spend the greater portion of his time in the open air, still more, his surroundings were such that if a lover of nature or of sport, he necessarily forgot himself, and thus was nature aided, and vigor and health restored. I have long been convinced that the most important factor in the successful management of pulmonary tuberculosis is to be found in climate (*Medical Record,* vol. 15, April 26, 1879, p. 387).

Loomis's explanation of the pure air followed.

The elevation of this region, its sandy soil, the undulating nature of the country, which ensures perfect drainage; the absence of cultivation, even of dwellings—all these conditions preclude the presence of telluric or miasmatic poison, and we have a purity of atmosphere unknown in more settled districts. The forests of this region are almost unbroken, stretching over the valleys, covering the mountains often to their very summit, and extending in some directions for nearly a hundred miles, while innumerable lakes dot this elevated plateau, and give moisture to the air. That the atmosphere of such a region, especially when set in motion, should by its contact with myriads of tree-tops and pine sheaves, become heavily laden with ozone is a natural sequence. Whatever other properties this gas may hereafter be found to possess, we know that it is a powerful disinfectant and Nature's choice agent for counteracting atmospheric impurities. . . . Pine, balsam, spruce, and hemlock trees abound, and the air is heavily laden with the resinous odors which they exhale. An agent which it is universally admitted exerts a most beneficial influence on diseased mucous membranes is thus brought in contact with the air-passages, while balsamics, which are also disinfectants, purify the atmosphere, which is constantly impregnated with them. Besides this, the air of the wilderness is optically pure, noticeably free from dust or visible particles of any kind. The invalid, therefore, is here surrounded by a zone of pure air, which separates him, as it were, from the germ pervaded world, and his diseased lungs are supplied with a specially vitalized and purified atmosphere, free from germs and impurities of any kind, and laden with the resinous exhalations of myriads of evergreens. (*Medical Record,* vol. 15, April 26, 1879, pp. 386–87).

With some provincial pride Loomis quoted Dr. Trudeau's letter, "My own personal experience and my personal observation of other phthisical invalids lead me to say that any comparison of the relative good effects of the climate of St. Paul, Minn., or of the South, with that of the Adirondack region is decidedly in favor of the latter." Another quote from the letter described Trudeau's personal experience with the Adirondack guides' cure in the area:

Camping out, which is the peculiar feature of this place . . . from June to October. I consider an important and beneficial measure in the treatment of phthisis. . . . The advantages gained by this mode of life are evident. The phthisical invalid for four months, night and day, lives out-of-doors, in a pure atmosphere; he is quiet, has perfect rest, plenty of good food (for which this mode of life gives an amazing relish); he has no opportunity to daily observe the effect upon other phthisical invalids of the disease from which he is suffering; his surroundings are such that he can lie down whenever standing fatigues him, can eat whenever he is hungry, sleep when exhausted, and dress as suits his own comfort—all of which comforts the requirements of society sometimes interfere with.

All these things—the breathing of the pure air of the wilderness, the perfect rest, the wholesome food, and early hours—combine to make tent-life a powerful weapon in combating this disease (*Medical Record,* vol. 15, April 26, 1879, p. 387).

Trudeau may not have realized that not everyone would find "camping out" as rewarding as he did, but certainly it provided him with a completely relaxing and enjoyable experience. However it was not inexpensive and required the services of a full-time wilderness guide who provided all of the comforts that the invalid enjoyed. Loomis then described twenty cases, concluding: "Of the twenty persons who have tested the therapeutical power of the climate of the Adirondack region by giving it an extended trial, ten have recovered, six have been improved, two have not been benefited, and two have died" (*Medical Journal*, vol. 15, May 3, 1879, p. 412).

This paper advertised the Adirondack region as a climate suitable for curing consumption. Dr. Loomis's agent in the area was Edward Trudeau, who supervised cases while Loomis was in New York City. This must have given Trudeau some hope that there was a market for his services similar to what existed at other popular cure centers in South Carolina, Minnesota, New Mexico, and Colorado. Both Loomis and Trudeau were living proof that the Adirondack climate had made a difference. Confirmation of their belief in the healing woods existed.

MEDICAL COMPETITION OVER CLIMATE

That climate was a popular topic is reflected by a discussion in May 1879 at the annual AMA meeting in Atlanta of "sanitaria for the treatment of pulmonary phthisis with special emphasis upon Alpine sanitaria" (*Medical Record,* vol. 15, May 17, 1879, p. 471).

Not to be outdone by a New Yorker, Dr. W. H. Geddings began the first of many annual reports of cases who had benefited from the climate of Aiken, South Carolina: "The publication in *Medical Record* last spring, by Prof. Loomis, of a few cases [note his emphasis] successfully treated in the Adirondack Region, determined the writer to carry out a resolution made several years ago, to publish each year the results of all cases of consumption that came under his observation in the course of the season."

After describing thirty-one cases for the "season 1878–79" Geddings concluded,

It will be seen by the table, that nineteen out of thirty-one cases were more or less improved, that in four of these there was entire cessation of cough, the patients being to all appearances quite well when they left Aiken. . . . A fact worthy of note . . . is that patients wintering at Aiken, as a rule, did better than those which did not arrive until after the warm weather of spring had begun (*Medical Record,* vol. 16, November 15, 1879, pp. 461–66).

Additional reports were made for the seasons 1879–80 (vol. 18, October 30, 1880, pp. 513–18), 1880–81 (vol. 21, January 7, 1882) and through 1885.

Another North Carolinian, Dr. Edwin A. Gatchell argued that his region, Asheville in Buncombe County, enjoyed a "wide reputation as a resort for the cure of incipient phthisis." Gatchell's testimony was supported by testimonials from other local physicians (*Medical Record,* vol. 26, September 27, 1884, p. 364).

Not to be outdone by the eastern doctors, Dr. Talbot Jones of St. Paul, Minnesota, presented cases of tuberculous patients who had spent the winter, commenting:

The cases I herewith report will show that, far from being injurious, the winter climate of the State is positively curative or beneficial. I place these cases, without comment, before the profession, and allow them to draw their own deductions as to the result. I need scarcely say that they are not selected ones . . . and none have been withheld from publication on account of being unfavorable cases for a report. This is too serious a subject to be treated in any such spirit of bias or prejudice. That which is desirable in the study of this subject, to learn, and which it is of the utmost importance to know, is the actual effects of cold climates and warm upon phthisis; and having ascertained this, we can then exercise a wise determination in the selection of a climate which will be best adapted to each individual case (*Medical Record,* vol. 17, March 6, 1880, pp. 252–55).

One wonders how Trudeau reacted to these claims for a particular region. Did he suspect the data might be biased, as Dr. Jones implied? Did he question the data based on the fact that he had not done well at Aiken during the spring of 1873 or St. Paul in the winter of 1873–74? Or did he reconcile his own experience with these competing reports by agreeing with Shrady's editorial in the fall of 1880? Aware that several climates claimed to be superior, including the Adirondacks, Shrady argued,

There is undoubtedly a best place for each case of phthisis; and there is not any ideal spot as yet known which meets all conditions and is suitable for all phases of the disease. The problem is to fit the proper climate to the patient. . . . We can only say now that probably dryness, purity, coolness, and equability meet the most indications, but that atmospheric rarity, coldness, warmth, ozone, electricity, balsamic odors, and various local conditions or personal idiosyncrasies, must often be given a high prominence in the selection of the best climate for a particular case of phthisis (*Medical Record,* vol. 18, November 13, 1880, p. 547).

Shrady's editorial is a beautiful illustration of the notion of "specificity," which became popular in the 1860s. It reflected the general notion that "change of climate" implied removal from the poverty and filth of cities, which the wealthy could avoid. Also it neatly paraphrased a July article, "On the Treatment of Various Forms of Consumption," by Professor Robert Bartholow, who recommended "a climate possessing purity, dryness, elevation, and uniform moisture and temperature is best for consumptives with proper care to hygiene and nutrition" (*American Journal of Medical Science*, vol. 80, July 1880, p. 255). Shrady recognized that there was a scientific methodology that could decide the question once the necessary data became available. "We can conclude from all this that there is as yet neither sufficient physiological knowledge or statistical evidence to settle definitely the true value of high altitudes" (*Medical Record,* vol. 18, November 13, 1880, p. 546).

Clearly, he did not want to allow physicians to settle the issue on the basis of clinical experience and professional testimonials. This is particularly obvious in Shrady's comment on a committee report of the California State Board of Health for 1880, which had been authorized by the State Legislature "to investigate the subject of a suitable locality for a State hospital for consumptives." Ten sites were investigated using the following criteria: "a certain equability of temperature, the absence of excessive humidity, elevation, exemption from fogs and strong winds, an abundant supply of pure water, and opportunities for a pleasant out-door life, either of work or recreation."

The committee selected two sites, the Sierra Madre Villa in Los Angeles County and Atlas Peak in Napa County. Shrady's comment reveals his scientific concern and probably an eastern bias:

The opinions expressed in this report in question are based in many instances on somewhat meager data. Even in the case of the Atlas Peak country there are no definite facts given regarding the actual effect of the climate upon phthisical patients. Neither do we find in the report any special preference to the character of the soil, except as regards its fertility. Notwithstanding this incompleteness, however, the report is a most instructive one, on account of the very frank and unbiased manner in which it discusses the value of the different health resorts. It will show the reader where he will be likely to find the most healthful locality for consumptives. It will also show him that California possesses no sanitaria, so far as is known, which have any remarkable power in checking or curing pulmonary disease (*Medical Record*, vol. 19, March 19, 1881, pp. 322–23).

Shrady wanted physicians to make decisions on more than opinion and testimonials. Epidemiological data would become necessary for medical decision making.

In "Medical Items and News" in October 1881, the *Medical Record*, carried a negative report on Trudeau's territory called "Consumptives in the Adirondacks":

Two or three deaths from consumption are reported from the region near Lake Placid within a week. Through the summer [1881] nineteen deaths are reported throughout the Adirondack region among the cases sent there to benefit. This mortality is probably caused by the great dampness near the lakes, the violent changes of temperature peculiar to the country, and the poor nourishment usually obtained in the houses and camps. Only a few found relief from this disease in those mountains (*Medical Record*, vol. 20, October 1, 1881, p. 387).

That report was tempered somewhat by an editorial four weeks later on "The Adirondack Cure for Phthisis": "Under the stimulus of an ill-advised magazine article, the Adirondack region was widely invaded by phthisical patients last summer. We now hear from all sides complaints that very little good was effected there; that many persons died in the woods; and that many others received absolutely no benefit. The impression is abroad that the 'wilderness cure' is a failure."

An article, "The Wilderness Cure," had been written by Marc Cook and published in 1881 by Wm. Woods and Company, the publisher of the *Medical Record*. Shrady then reminded his readers of the notion of "specificity," referring to Dr. Loomis's 1879 article on "The Adirondack Region as a Therapeutical Agent in the Treatment of Pulmonary Phthisis."

Dr. Loomis's observation tended to show that it was in certain forms of catarrhal phthisis that benefit or cure was to be expected. Fibrous phthisis would, he thought, do better in Colorado. Tubercular phthisis and some of the catarrhal forms could not be expected to improve anywhere.

Now this presentation of the wilderness cure is very different from that of the enthusiastic, but very unwise gentleman, who, having cured himself in the Adirondacks, "wrote up the wilderness in glowing colors."

It is no wonder that many bitter disappointments followed to those who caught the hopeful spirit of the book's work. Perhaps even medical men were a little affected by it. Otherwise, it does not seem possible to explain the many phthisical invalids, entirely unfit for camp life anywhere who swarmed into the St. Regis region, there to die. . . . The wilderness cure has not yet proved a failure, but it is proved that the class of cases who may be benefited there must be carefully selected ones. . . .

We may in time learn that the Adirondacks are no better than almost any other mountain resorts; but definite opinions must be based in statistics not yet obtainable. . . .

It may be well to remember, however, that cold and high altitudes for phthisis are just now in fashion (*Medical Record,* vol. 20, October 29, 1881, pp. 490–91).

The question of the climate for the cure of phthisis would go on but Shrady at least had made two points: (1) that "data," not "testimonials," should be used to decide the question and (2) that certain cases might benefit from certain climates ("specificity"). To answer these questions an experiment was required. Both Loomis and Trudeau, two arrested consumptives partial to the Adirondacks, were in an ideal position in 1882 to attempt one.

TREATING PATIENTS IN THE WOODS

But how would he treat patients? Two approaches were available from Trudeau's training and the medical literature of the time. First, the knowledge that tuberculosis was "self-limiting," that people could recover spontaneously from tuberculosis, suggested a holistic approach. This involved removing the patient from the environment that produced tuberculosis, thereby reducing the stressful social situation and avoiding exposure to a noxious workplace. Then effort could be focused on building up the body by good nutrition and rest.

Second, the local lesion would be treated. Cough, hemoptysis (spitting blood), night sweats, wasting (weight loss), and cavities in the lung could be treated by specific remedies from the physician's arsenal of drugs. Often the two approaches were combined.

General Health and Nutrition

Reviewing the third edition, in 1879, of *On the Treatment of Pulmonary Consumption* by J. H. Bennett, M.D., Shrady said that the author "directs the attention of the profession to the general health and nutrition of the patient rather than the local lesion" and remarks that the value of this advice is currently well recognized (*Medical Record,* vol. 15, April 5, 1879, p. 329).

In the discussion that followed Dr. Austin Flint's paper on "Self-limitation in Cases of Phthisis" before the New York Academy of Medicine, Dr. J. R. Leaming stated that "the office of the physician should be to assist nature" by removing the irritating agent and providing good nutrition (*Medical Record,* vol. 16, July 19, 1879, p. 67). Similar statements were made by Prof. Bartholow (*American Journal of Medical Sciences,* vol. 80, July 1880, p. 255).

This seemed to be the accepted general method of treatment from 1879 to 1882, as Shrady implied when he summarized an original communication on "Early Indications of Phthisis" sent by Dr. William Porter of St. Louis,

in which he does not state anything new, but rather enforces the necessity of early recognizing the initial lesions of the disease, and of using proper means for their relief or cure . . . the remaining salient points . . . relative to treatment are as follows:
1. Thorough protection of the body from injurious atmospheric or telluric influences.
2. Correction of a faulty condition of the digestive organs, for the purpose of securing a proper assimilation of nutritious food.   3. Early removal of the patient to a climate which will tend to invigorate the physical forces. It is certainly true that these rules, when strictly observed, are productive of greater benefit to the patient than hyper-medication (*Medical Record,* vol. 21, February 25, 1882, p. 205).

Such a treatment would have been completely compatible with Trudeau's cure experience with the Adirondack guides during his stays at Paul Smith's. Despite repeated attempts, the social and environmental atmosphere of Manhattan was not something his body could tolerate.

But while he retreated to the wilderness to rest under the trees and look out on the lake his strength and appetite slowly returned (Trudeau, 1915, p. 98). This form of treatment did not provide much of a role for the physician. In fact, Trudeau's caregivers had been guides like Warren Flanders, who knew how to cater to wealthy sportsmen and invalids. If the physician merely catered to the general health and nutrition of the patient, the caregiving role was reduced to that of a hotelier or wilderness guide. And how could one tell whether the patient's recovery had been spontaneous because the disease was self-limiting, or had been due to an improvement in general health and nutrition? This question always concerned Trudeau. Despite the fact that such care may have been all that was necessary, Trudeau and other physicians found a role by treating the various symptoms of tuberculosis.

Treating Symptoms

Probably one of the easiest symptoms to treat was "loss of appetite." Porter called it "correction of a faulty condition of the digestive organ." No doubt many tuberculous patients, removed from jobs in noxious factories, forced to rest, and served nutritious food, regained their appetites in time. But physicians felt this process could be accelerated.

It was felt that tonics and other substances such as "chloride of ammonium, cod-liver oil, quinine" could stimulate the appetite (*Medical Record,* vol. 15, May 3, 1879, p. 427). Shrady reported on an article from the *Lancet* of September 6, 1879, in which patients were given hypophosphites ("eight grams each of the hypophosphite of soda and lime in an ounce of the infusion of cascarilla, . . . twice a day after meals"). "It was considered proved by a comparison of the cases that the hypophosphites have no claim to be considered a specific remedy for phthisis. They have, however, valuable tonic properties, improving the appetite, increasing the weight, and helping digestion" (*Medical Record,* vol. 16, October 11, 1879, p. 348).

Cod-liver oil seemed to have been an important nutritional supplement. Beverley Robinson, M.D., lecturer on Clinical Medicine at Bellevue Hospital Medical College, described the case of a seventeen-year-old printer with cough, spitting of blood, and loss of weight.

Of course I shall keep this boy on an emulsion of cod-liver oil, and I will also deem it indicated to place repeated fly-blisters under his clavicles to diminish localized congestion, due to whatever cause it may be. . . .

If haemoptysis [spitting blood] continues . . . I shall . . . advise regular habits, restraint from over-muscular exercise of any and all descriptions, denial of all stimulants, such as tea, coffee, and alcohol. This boy should live a great deal in the open air, and eat abundantly of azotized food [charged with nitrogen] (*Medical Record,* vol. 17, January 31, 1880, pp. 112–13).

Physicians in 1879 and 1880 were developing a role for themselves by caring for the symptoms of tuberculous patients. The four-part treatment recommended by Carl Both, M.D., in an "Original Communication" systematized the doctor's intervention. It involved

1. The cleansing of the bronchi of mucus and pus, and afterward the normal expansion of the air-vesicles by means of actively exercising the respiratory muscles.

2. The careful study of the needs of the system for certain articles of food containing lime salts; and a proper appreciation of the necessity of getting rid of excrementitious substances as quickly as possible.

3. In a medication of certain minerals in organic form, such as lime and silica, for the purpose of aiding the calcification of tubercles; and in acids such as citric, which contain an excess of oxygen, and which tend to help oxidation of protein substances.

4. In bringing the patient in such condition of life that his nervous system is not unnecessarily overtaxed at the same time it is so employed as to balance nervous force and stimulate his general nutrition as much as possible (*Medical Record,* vol. 18, February 21, 1880, pp. 200–203).

Though this procedure appears to be written to impress the reader, the treatment is not that different from caring for the general health and nutrition except that it gives the physician something to do in the role of monitor or supervisor. Incidentally, as Dr. Both was one of the few physicians who had his address printed in the journal, one wonders if the article wasn't a subtle form of advertisement, as he reported on cases he had presented in 1878 and added new cases, arguing that phthisis was curable. "These cases must convince the most conservative sceptic that tuberculosis of the lungs can be arrested to a degree heretofore considered absolutely impossible" (*Medical Record,* vol. 17, February 21, 1880, p. 203).

Finally Shrady reported in an editorial that force-feeding of phthisical patients achieved good results. Weight is gained rapidly. Cough and spitting diminish and the lungs begin to repair, but the report does not give evidence of permanent cures. Presumably, force-feeding can be a medical procedure, while normal eating of nutritious food might be done without medical supervision (*Medical Record,* vol. 22, December 30, 1881, p. 739).

Cough

Cough and expectoration of a yellow pus-like sputum or phlegm sometimes with blood (haemoptysis) were treated with a variety of remedies. Reporting an address given at the British Medical Association, Dr. Andrew Clark advocated giving antimony in "doses of 1/25th of a grain every hour" to relieve the condition of bronchitis that affects many tuberculosis patients have (*Medical Record,* vol. 16, September 13, 1879, p. 255). When spitting of blood continues, Dr. Beverly Robinson recommended frequently repeated doses of ergot, a drug commonly used to control bleeding such as hemorrhage after giving birth (*Medical Record,* vol. 17, January 31, 1880, p. 113).

Shrady reported the relief of cough by the hypodermic injection of water by Prof. Landouzy in France:

The injection may be made at the neck, near the larynyx, in the infraclavicular region, or in an intercoastal space, accordingly as the patient points out one or another of the localities as the starting point of the irritation. It appears to be of some importance to hide the nature of the fluid from the patient's knowledge, and for this reason a few drops of aqua laurocerasi may be added to the water (*Medical Record,* vol. 14, January 29, 1881, p. 121).

One wonders whether the claimed relief was due to the water or to the placebo effect. Though treatment of cough may not have been essential, in many cases it would make patients more comfortable, allowing them to sleep and regain their strength.

Fever

Fever was a common symptom of tuberculosis made more significant by the fact that it could now be measured quite accurately by using a thermometer. It occurred daily, often increasing in the evening and producing night sweats. From the *Practitioner* of December 1879 came the results of a Dr. Murrell, who treated thirty-three cases of sweating, of whom thirty were phthisical patients, with jaborandi and pilocarpine. [Jaborandi is the leaf of a South American shrub that produces salivation, sweating, increased flow of the secretions, and lowering of temperature and blood pressure. Pilocarpine is a salt derived from jaborandi.] "Phthisical patients stated that the drug 'did the cough good, brought up the phlegm,' and 'eased the breathing.' It is therefore useful as an expectorant" (*Medical Record,* vol. 17, March 6, 1880, p. 259).

The next week another treatment for night sweats was reported:

Dr. Kohnhorn reports two cases which had resisted the successive employment of quinine, atropia, digitalis, boletus, caricis, folia salviae, and various external lavements, frictions, inunctions, etc. These cases were quickly cured by the external application of a powder prepared using acid salicyl, anayl, and talc. . . . The entire surface of the body is powdered over (*Medical Record,* vol. 17, March 13, 1880, p. 287).

And two years later Shrady reported an alternative to a commonly used drug, atropin:

Dr. Froumuller reports sixteen cases of phthisis with night-sweats in which homatropin was successfully used. . . . It was found that one injection would stop the night sweats for several days. The fever and cough were also lessened and the drug seemed to have the effect of bringing the disease to a standstill for a time. The advantage over atropin is that it (homatropin) produces its effects without any toxic symptoms, such as widening of the pupil, dryness of the throat, etc. (*Medical Record,* vol. 21, April 22, 1882, p. 437).

The symptoms of cough and fever had been treated by physicians for many years. Back in 1861 Alonzo Clark recommended to students at the College of

Physicians and Surgeons that they must first "build up" the patient with the best food and tonics. He strongly prescribed cod-liver oil for contributing to the general health and nutrition of the patient (Purdy, 1890).

Clark cautioned his students to remember that cough may be necessary to remove fluids but that if it became too severe they could use Balsam tolu [a resin from *Toluifera balsamum*, a tree of tropical America] in ipecac [the dried rhizome and roots of *Cephaelis ipecacunha* or of *Cephaelis acuminata*, rubiaceous plants of tropical America used in small doses for laryngitis and bronchitis]. If the patient needed to be relaxed, opium or morphine might be used or even Ayers Cherry Pectoral, a "quack medicine" containing tartar of antimony (Purdy, 1890).

For haemoptysis (coughing blood) it was thought that the patient should be quieted down with a placebo or opium if necessary. Night sweats could be treated with quinine and excess of Elixir of Vitriol or rubbing the body with alcohol if necessary (Purdy, 1890).

Although Shrady's journal reported some newer treatments for these symptoms, they are not mentioned as remarkable discoveries and in many cases the reader is not even encouraged to try them. It is likely that Trudeau had been treating these common symptoms during his brief professional career and likely followed the commonly accepted practices recommended by Alonzo Clark. However, there was one treatment that Clark had not mentioned. It appears to have become popular in 1879 and Shrady mentioned it frequently in 1880, 1881, and 1882.

Inhalation Therapy

Inhalation was an accepted form of treatment by 1882. The question was, what substance should the patient inhale? If Trudeau followed Shrady's suggestion, creosote or carbolic acid seemed to show the greatest promise. However, a number of different substances were used and described in the medical literature of the time.

In England, where Lister had first developed the atomizer for directing a fine spray of carbolic acid onto surgical sites, antiseptic respirators were used, and different models were available (*Medical Record*, vol. 20, December 24, 1881, p. 709). The reader will remember that Lister had visited the United States in 1876, arguing that carbolic acid should be used as an antiseptic spray to kill bacteria on surgical sites. It was not very different to argue that bacteria on an interior cavity such as the lung could be killed by inhaling carbolic acid. This idea was expressed by F. H. Devis, M.D., of Chicago and quoted from the *Detroit Lancet* of May 1879. He used inhalation in the treatment of pulmonary diseases such as chronic bronchitis. "Inhalation of steam impregnated with the vapor of carbolic acid and camph. tincture of opium will be found to afford prompt relief to all of the immediate symptoms, the carbolic acid acting as an antiseptic, while the moist warmth and the opiates allay local irritation and the resulting cough" (*Medical Record*, vol. 15, June 7, 1879, pp. 551–52). Dr. J. M. Dacosta at the Pennsylvania Hospital in Philadelphia had reported using "inhalations of carbolic acid" on a thirty-one-year-old sailor with pulmonary disease (*Medical Record,* vol. 8, April 20, 1878, p. 330).

While the Americans reported individual clinical cases, Shrady looked to Europe for solid evidence that inhalation was effective and reported the following in "Medical Items and News" under the title "The Cure of Consumption":

There seems to be grounds at last for hoping that a really effective curative agent against consumption in all its forms has been found. Professor Klebs, of Munich, some time ago, calling attention to the large number of internal diseases known to be caused by infection, classed them among the tubercular diseases. Dr. Max Schneller of Greifswald, being interested in the subject tried several experiments, and having produced tuberculosis in two groups of rabbits, subjected one group to the ordinary treatment, and put the other for several hours daily "in a box filled with vapor of a solution of what the Germans call 'benzoesaures Natron.' " The former group died, the latter recovered perfect health. Professor Rokitansky has since tried making his consumptives at Innsbruck inhale similar vapors daily. The results are said to have "far surpassed his hopes," and high medical authorities are of the opinion that at last a real advance has been made in solving one of the most important and difficult of modern medical problems (*Medical Record,* vol. 18, January 24, 1880, p. 107).

Two issues later Shrady described Rokitansky's method in the "Progress of Medical Science" section under the title "Inhalations of Benzoate of Soda":

Rokitansky makes his patients inhale daily one gramme of the drug (in a five percent solution) for every $2\frac{1}{2}$ pounds of their weight. He attributes to this medication, first of all, a destructive action on bacteria; and secondly, a mechanical action on the pathological secretions, which are rendered more liquid and are more readily removed from the air passages. This results in an amelioration of the catarrhal symptoms, and perhaps prevents the transformation of the secretions into caseous masses. Further, he believes that the forced inspirations and expirations dilate the air-vesicles by interalveolar tubercular masses. He is convinced, moreover, that the benzoate of soda, when used in this manner for a long time, acts as a febrifuge. Of course, he combines with the inhalations the usual hygienic and dietetic treatment (*Medical Record,* vol. 17, February 7, 1880, p. 147).

In the same article Shrady presented a criticism:

Dr. Schnitzler of Vienna, on the other hand, is inclined to be skeptical with regard to the value of these inhalations. For the sake of experiment, he made a large number of patients inhale a five per cent solution of benzoate of soda, which had been colored with a few drops of aniline, or alternately solutions of tannin and perchloride of iron, and, on examining them afterward with the laryngoscope, found the mouth and pharynx uniformly discolored by the solutions, while the larynx and trachea presented only a few isolated discolored spots. From this he argues that atomized liquids do not penetrate to any extent into the bronchi and that the marvelous effects attributed to the benzoate of soda, if not entirely illusive, must be ascribed to the volatilization by heat of the benzoic acid, which can then undoubtedly penetrate into the smallest tubes. Hence, he claims that it would be more logical to employ directly the volatile benzoic acid for the inhalations, and that if any special curative action be expected from the benzoate of soda, it would be preferable to administer it internally, when the same result could be obtained with much smaller doses. He closes his paper by recommending, as an antiparasitic treatment of phthisis, the inhalation and subcutaneous injection of carbolic acid, a treatment that he has employed for three years with relatively very favorable results (*Medical Record,* vol. 17, February 7, 1880, p. 147).

This is an interesting example of knowledge developing. Rokitansky explained his successful results by claiming the inhalations reached the bacteria in the lungs. Schnitzler tested this claim by coloring the inhaled vapor and discovered it hardly reached the larynx and trachea, concluding it was unlikely to penetrate to the lungs. Rather than use a diluted solution of benzoate of soda, Schnitzler argued for the volatile form of benzoic acid or carbolic acid in order to penetrate into the lungs. None of these studies used control groups of patients who were not treated. Their claim to effectiveness is based on the observation and testimony of the treating physician.

About a month and a half later, in the "Progress" section, Shrady quoted from a letter written to a German journal by Klebs:

Prof. Klebs, . . . gives the results of a series of investigations with the following conclusions: tuberculosis, miliary eruptions can be made to proceed to self limitation or retrogression by the internal administration of the benzoates, particularly the benzoate of magnesia. . . . In apex infiltrations, unless of very long standing, even when accompanied by hectic fever and preceded by haemoptysis, the exclusive application of soda benzoates by inhalation (grm. 10 a day), or by insufflation (grm. 2–3 a day) together with the internal administration of benzoate of magnesia, accomplishes a permanent lowering of temperature, cessation of catarrhal manifestations, and increase of the bodily weight (*Medical Record,* vol. 17, March 20, 1880, p. 316).

Having presented several articles on inhalation, Shrady wrote a cautious summary editorial called "The Benzoate of Soda in Phthisis":

Within the past six months considerable attention has been directed to the benzoate of sodium as a remedy for phthisis. Although the profession naturally looks with distrust upon any agent said to have a curative agency in tubercular disease, the strong advocacy of the claims of the salt in question by several leading men has invited serious discussion. From time to time we have noticed the reports, mainly from foreign sources, concerning the so-called efficiency of this drug. As might have been expected, the accounts of the results obtained are somewhat exaggerated and conflicting. The very hope that phthisis can be cured by a single remedy is enough to pardon the enthusiasm which has been infused into the discussion of the subject. It is hard to believe that the salt has any special effect upon the disease. We cannot afford, however, to ignore the statements of men who have good reputations, who are competent observers and conscientious practitioners.

Shrady reviewed the history of the use of benzoate of soda, mentioning nine practitioners who reported positive results and three who reported negative or "injurious effects of these inhalations." Then he described a consensus conference. "At Innsbruck a special committee of competent medical men was appointed for the purpose of investigating this subject. The report of this committee was quite unfavorable to the general utility of these inhalations in phthisis." Following this report, Shrady made his judgment.

From these brief abstracts of the most important publications on this subject we are unable to deduce any convincing proof of the real value of this, the latest anti-phthisical remedy. Still it is quite evident that the benzoates had an extended trial. . . . If experience realizes a tithe of the expectations which are entertained of its curative properties in phthisis, the profession can take courage in still fighting against the odds in this disease, and taking the chances for success, desperate as they are (*Medical Record,* vol. 17, March 27, 1880, pp. 349–50).

Shrady's remarks are almost those of a coach or teacher saying, that was a good try, you scientists. Tuberculosis is still out there as our challenge, keep up the good fight. We have no way of knowing whether Trudeau read these *Medical Record* articles and editorials, but Shrady felt that these European scientists and practitioners were the source of hope in the fight against tuberculosis.

In the next issue he listed more negative results by two Berlin physicians, Guttmann in thirty-one cases, and Wenzel in ten cases (*Medical Record,* vol. 17, April 3, 1880, p. 373). Having pretty well eliminated benzoate of soda, Shrady reported a new wrinkle in inhalation therapy using borax and salicylic acid. Dr. Sachse of Berlin reported "remarkable success" using "750 parts water, 25 parts salicylic acid, 19½ parts borax" in morning and evening inhalations for five or ten minutes (*Medical Record,* vol. 17, May 29, 1880, p. 590). Inhalation still seemed to be an acceptable form of treatment; the problem was, what was the appropriate substance to be inhaled?

A year later Shrady reported encouraging results:

Dr. G. Hunter Mackenzie records in detail the successful treatment of a case of acute phthisis by causing the patient to respire as continuously as possible an "antiseptic" atmosphere. The results obtained would appear to bear out the experiments of Schuler and Griefswald, who found that animals rendered artificially tuberculous were cured by being made to inhale creosote water for lengthened periods.

The patient was an eighteen-year-old, who had been sent to the country and given cod-liver oil with hypophosphites and an "abundance of milk," which did not relieve his condition. He was then treated by inhalation of an "antiseptic atmosphere," which resulted in "1. slight fall of temperature; 2. great diminution of the cough with complete cessation of the muco-purulent sputum; 3. marked improvement in the appetite and general strength; 4. gradual abolition of the night sweats; 5. improvement in the physical condition of the lungs." Commenting on these positive results, Shrady said that Dr. Mackenzie uses

various volatile antiseptics such as creosote, carbolic acid, and thymol; the latter he has discarded as being too irritating and inefficient. Carbolic acid seems to be absorbed, for it has been detected freely in the urine; no trace of creosote . . . has been found. . . . An absorption of the particular drug employed is not deemed necessary, and therefore not to be desired, he now uses creosote only, either pure or dissolved in one to three parts of rectified spirit. Whether the success as far attained is due to the antidotal action of creosote and carbolic acid on a specific tubercular neoplasm, or to their action as preventives of septic poisoning from the local centers in the lungs, it is certain that their continuous, steady use in the manner described has a decidedly curative action in acute phthisis, and is therefore worthy of an extended trial (*Medical Record,* vol. 20, July 9, 1881, p. 41).

That Shrady reported this one case with such positive enthusiasm or hope is evidence that clinical cases without controls, when presented in a "scientific" way (e.g., with urine analysis) by a reputable practitioner, could be convincing in 1881. Sanctioned by the eminent editor of the *Medical Record,* the case no doubt carried considerable authority.

Other substances were suggested as inhalants,

In laryngeal phthisis, says Dr. Bird (*Australian Medical Journal*), an inhalation, with Siegle's spray, of filtered solution of hydrastin, with glycerine of borax and morphia, gives great temporary relief (*Medical Record,* vol. 21, January 14, 1882, p. 56).

Dr. B. Kussner, of Halle, argues for long term inhalation of iodoform in cure of phthisis. . . . We fear, however, that many persons will prefer phthisis to constantly inhaling iodoform, even if that drug proved of decided value (*Medical Record,* vol. 22, July 15, 1882, p. 70).

Mr. H. Osborn Bayfield suggests that the use of inhalations of volatilized palm oil may be useful in the treatment of phthisis. He bases his opinion upon the fact that workmen engaged in tinning where palm oil is used as a flux inhale the volatilized oil and get fat. Those previously emaciated or weak, rapidly improve. The idea is worth a trial (from the *British Medical Journal* in the *Medical Record,* vol. 29, October 14, 1882, p. 447).

Herr Kircher, a pupil of Liebig, has been during forty-four years, director of an ultramarine factory in which a special process of manufacture is employed which involves the formation of sulphurous acid by the burning of sulphur. He maintains (according to the *Gesundheit*) that none of his work-people have ever suffered from consumption, typhus, cholera, or any disorder, which is produced by bacteria. He recommends the following treatment in the case of tuberculous patients. They should be brought into a room in which small quantities of sulphur (one to two drachmas) are burnt every hour over a spirit-lamp or on a stove. At first coughing of a more or less aggravated character takes place, and after eight or twelve days the bacteria gradually disappear and cease to irritate the lung tissue. To complete the cure, the patients should be brought into rooms which contain some aromatic vapors (*Medical Record,* vol. 23, February 17, 1882, p. 195).

Other Treatments

In addition to the treatments listed above, several others are mentioned in the *Medical Record*. It is difficult to know how much credibility the editor gave to these "cures." They rarely appeared under "Progress in Medical Science." In his desire to leave no stone unturned, perhaps he felt they should be mentioned. Or perhaps this is an example of the Jacksonian tolerance that respected the opinion of every professional until proven otherwise. The *Journal*'s editorial policy pledged to be impartial in reviewing books and, with regard to submissions of materials, "impartial to all, unjust to none" (*Medical Record,* vol. 1, March 1, 1866, p. 14). As the *Medical Record* was a publishing enterprise, acknowledging communication in print could have had the effect of increasing circulation. Some treatments were no doubt just amusing.

Physicians had favorite potions they used. One from a Virginia physician was called "phosphoric emulsion." It was made by combining oil of bitter almonds with a mixture of equal parts of glycerine and egg yolk to which was added pure cod-liver oil while stirring vigorously. To this emulsion was added dilute phosphoric acid and rum. One tablespoonful was given after each meal, apparently as a tonic (*Medical Record,* vol. 16, July 5, 1879, p. 24).

Not to be outdone was M. M. Griffin, M.D., of Bradford, Pennsylvania, who sent the *Medical Record* the following:

A great many "new remedies" and "new preparations" are now before the public for consideration and for sale. I would call attention to an old one. It is a well-known fact that consumption is almost unknown in the oil regions of Pennsylvania—and that it is never developed here. The only reason for it is that we are daily consuming more or less of it in the water we drink and use in cooking purposes. The water obtained from the best wells and other sources, if left over-night in an ordinary vessel will be covered in the morning with a scum of oil. It is evident that most of us consume more or less of it. Consumptive persons coming here from a distance soon find speedy relief from their lung difficulties, and rapidly gain flesh and strength. The climate of Bradford is the most unfavorable; the days in summer are very warm, the nights cold and damp, and the weather very changeable, and also much wet and disagreeable weather—so it cannot be the climate that effects the change. The crude petroleum no doubt, would long ago have become a popular remedy in lung difficulties if it had not been for its very nauseating properties. I have sent a supply of the crude oil of a semi-solid consistency, that accumulates on the sucker-rods and casings of the wells, which is readily prepared into pills by incorporating it with any inert vegetable powder, to a number of physicians and hospitals, with a request to give it a trial in their cases of consumption. Sufficient time had not elapsed to give a full report, but thus far the report has been very satisfactory. About fifty percent of cures are reported of acute phthisis. It afforded much relief in all curable cases. I do not claim that it is a specific, but that it will do more good in chronic lung troubles than anything yet suggested. The crude is rich in hydrocarbons, and seems to have a special action toward the lungs, relieving cough, hectic, night-sweats, and flesh and strength is rapidly gained. I have had it under trial now during the last twelve months and I can state that my faith in it grows stronger the oftener I prescribe it. . . . It is hoped that the profession will thoroughly investigate the matter and give their experience of this cheap and valuable medicine (*Medical Record,* vol. 16, October 11, 1879, p. 359).

Two years later, another physician from Bradford, M. Milton, wrote, "I am inclined to the opinion that in our great staple, crude petroleum oil, we have no mean means of alleviating or arresting the progress of this fatal malady. . . . I find the medicinal oil pleasant and palatable, and I think . . . it will become one of our most valuable medicines" (*Medical Record,* vol. 20, July 2, 1881, pp. 27–28).

Earlier in the century it was believed that people with strong lungs could be free of phthisis, and many were urged to exercise. Another version of this idea was reported by Shrady:

It is stated that, during the last twenty-five years, not a single singer at St. Petersburg has died of consumption although this disease has outstripped all others, and now holds the first place among the causes of death at the Russian capital. From this and other facts, Dr. Vasilieff draws an inference in favor of the exercise involved in singing, as a preventive measure against consumption. The Lancet, in quoting this conclusion, very properly warns the reader against adopting it too readily. It may either happen that singers are not consumptive, because they can use their throat and chest freely; or that consumptive persons are not singers, because the weakness that precedes disease incapacitates the chest and throat for exertion (*Medical Record,* vol. 16, December 6, 1879, p. 547).

Regardless of the value of this information, it does make an important methodological contribution, which Shrady chose to emphasize.

Hydrotherapy was mentioned as a treatment for consumption by a Professor Peter from Paris (*Medical Record,* vol. 18, August 7, 1880, p. 157). Dr. James Sawyer of Queens College, Birmingham, claimed

that he gets better results in treating phthisis by combining chloride of calcium with the standard remedies, than by any other means. He is inclined to place a high value on its curative effect. He thinks it checks night-sweats, increases weight and tends to dry up the lesions. He gives it in ten-grain doses, twice a day, after meals. There should be no mistake made by substituting chloride of "lime" for chloride of calcium (*Medical Record*, vol. 18, September 4, 1880, p. 252. Quoting from the *British Medical Journal*).

Dr. Ordylowski argued that chloral (a colorless, oily liquid, trichloracetic aldehyde, prepared by the mutual action of alcohol and chlorine) is useful in phthisis. It "relieves insomnia, diminishes night-sweats, checks somewhat the loss of weight, lowers the temperature, increases urinary secretion and improves the morale" (*Medical Record*, vol. 18, November 27, 1880, p. 603).

A somewhat more spectacular remedy was reported by Dr. John A. Wells as it was used on the service of Dr. Andrew H. Smith at Presbyterian Hospital in New York. Three cases are described. Archibald Sinclair, a twenty-year-old in the third stage of catarrhal phthisis, was given an enema of defibrinated blood.

Four ounces of defibrinated bullock's blood, to which four grains of chloral hydrate had been added, were administered per rectum, at bedtime, in addition to the usual treatment. . . . After three weeks, during which the amount was reduced to two ounces, the rectum not tolerating the original amount, and adding opium (5 drops of tincture of opium/4 ounces of blood). . . . The patient experienced weight gain, change in appearance, improved appetite and continuous improving one month later (*Medical Record*, vol. 19, March 5, 1881, p. 262).

Maria Durnin and Edward Haggerty, who were similarly sick with phthisis, received similar treatments and were much improved. The editor made no comments about these cases, but we can wonder how the patient's improvement can be attributed to the enema alone when simultaneously they were receiving dietary supplement, rest, and removal from their previous environment as well.

One cure is reported by the editor for entertainment under the title, "A Curious Specific for Consumption." "A well-dressed and apparently intelligent woman appeared at the dog pound in the city the other day, and asked for the forequarter of a dog that had been drowned. She said that her sister had consumption, and that someone had told her the forequarter of a drowned dog made into a stew would cure the disease. She got the meat and went away contented" (*Medical Record*, vol. 20, September 10, 1881, p. 305). "In a recent clinical lecture (*Maryland Medical Journal*) Dr. William H. Thomson called attention to certain cases in which the cough of phthisis is entirely suspended. Such an event may occur when there is a drain upon the system in some direction, as when diarrhea or chronic suppuration, or large excretion of urine sets in" (*Medical Record*, vol. 20, July 9, 1881, p. 55).

Dr. Brookes D. Baker, government physician in S. Koma, Hawaii, wrote "I have found by experience that the vomiting in phthisis can be controlled, in some thoroughly, in others partially, by the ether spray on the back of the neck, doing it just before meals. In very bad cases I have used it on the stomach as well" (*Medical Record,* vol. 21, June 3, 1882, p. 611). How many of these other remedies were presented as serious medical contributions is not clear. But they do reveal that clinical opinions were very common. Shrady presented some of them as curiosities, some as humor, some to maintain circulation, and some to illustrate important methodological points.

By 1882, when Trudeau decided to begin his sanitarium, most physicians had discarded the belief that tuberculosis was always fatal. It was believed to be contagious and, if Robert Koch were correct, to be caused by the tuberculosis bacillus. While many clinicians could not accept the idea of a "germ," others like Trudeau soon wanted to learn the new laboratory techniques described in Koch's paper. Having mastered these techniques and replicated Koch's work by 1883–84, Trudeau added to his reputation as an expert diagnostician. Not only did he diagnose, he also treated. We have seen the plethora of general and specific treatments available in the literature. Which of these did he adopt? To answer this question we look to Trudeau's case records.

NOTES

1. Mary Hotaling (1991) has clarified the confusing usage of the words "sanitarium" and "sanitorium."

> When Trudeau founded the Adirondack Cottage Sanitarium in 1884, he used the term applied to all chronic care institutions; it was derived from the Latin "sanitas" meaning "health," which denotes a "healthy place," but implies no curative effect. It was replaced by the term "sanitorium" (derived from "sanare"—"to cure" or "to heal"), which means "a place of healing." When *Tuberculosis Hospital and Sanatorium Construction* by Thomas Spees Carrington, M.D., was published in 1914, only the Adirondack Cottage Sanitarium of all the institutions it surveyed was still using the obsolete spelling; the term was modernized when it was renamed "Trudeau Sanitorium" after its founder's death in 1915. In the *Autobiography* he wrote at the end of his life, Trudeau (or his editor) carefully preserved the distinction observed here: "sanatorium" is used unless the Adirondack Cottage Sanitarium, 1884–1915, specifically, is meant (Hotaling, 1991, note 21).

I will follow Hotaling's convention.

2. With the help of student assistants I have read articles indexed under phthisis, consumption, and tuberculosis to understand what "medical science" was presenting as the current knowledge. By using direct quotations I intend to convey the content and the general methods of reasoning and communicating medical knowledge during that time. To assume that my reading is similar to that of Trudeau would be naive. We can only guess which articles he would have read thoroughly and which he ignored. Presumably he read articles by his friends and acquaintances. Thus I have paid special attention to articles written by New York City physicians, especially those associated with the College of Physicians and Surgeons.

Also, I have assumed that Trudeau paid special attention to articles by members of the American Climatological Association, which was founded in 1884 by his colleague and mentor Dr. A. L. Loomis. Beginning with forty-two charter members, the Association included seventy-four members by 1885, when Trudeau was admitted. This association was dedicated "to the study of climatology and the diseases of the respiratory organs." Originally limited to 100 active members who "had to deliver a paper" and could be rejected by "three black balls," the members of this organization appear to dominate the study of tuberculosis throughout Trudeau's lifetime (*Transactions of the American Climatological Association*, vol. 1, p. 5). The first president was A. L. Loomis, and W. H. Geddings (whom Trudeau must have met when he went to Aiken, South Carolina) was the second vice president. On the council were Beverly Robinson and Frank Donaldson, and members included well-known physicians like Shattuck, Kretzschmer, Dennison, Bosworth, Flint, and Leaming. By 1887 the association had appointed a special committee to assess the advantages and disadvantages of different health resorts at different altitudes and regions (*Transactions of the American Climatological Association*, vol. 4, Presidential Address, pp. 1–23).

6

Deciding How to Treat Patients

By 1879 Trudeau's health had improved and his expanding practice had convinced him that he could stay in the Adirondacks. One of the reasons the practice grew was his friend, colleague, and fellow consumptive, Dr. Alfred Loomis. Loomis had examined Trudeau each fall for five years and was impressed by his patient's improvement, so much so that he gave an enthusiastic paper to the Medical Society of the State of New York (*Medical Record,* vol. 15, nos. 17 and 18, April 26 and May 3, 1879, pp. 385–89, 409–12).

Loomis was a founder of the American Climatological Society, an organization of physicians devoted to studying the relation of climate to health. This recommendation of the Adirondack region from a leading medical practitioner gave hope to doctors in New York and elsewhere that something might be done for tuberculosis patients. Ordinarily their cases were considered hopelessly fatal.

Loomis's 1879 speech reflected a general groundswell of public sentiment regarding the healing attributes of nature. Beginning about 1840, enthusiastic vacationers had explored the Adirondacks, usually going west from Plattsburgh, Port Kent, or Westport on Lake Champlain. By 1856 Saranac Lake was "a settlement of fifteen scattered families." A series of hotels and hunting camps developed along the canoe and guide-boat routes. Martin's Hotel at the village of Saranac Lake on Lower Saranac Lake was built in the early 1850s and could accommodate 250 guests. Built in 1859, Paul Smith's St. Regis House on Lower St. Regis accommodated 100 guests. At the outlet between Upper Saranac Lake and Round Lake (Middle Saranac Lake), now known as Bartlett's Cary, was

Bartlett's, with rooms for fifty people, opened in the mid-1850s. At the southern end of Upper Saranac Lake was Jesse Corey's Rustic Lodge. Going south on Indian Carry (across Route 3, today) to Stoney Creek Ponds (Spectacle Ponds), one could reach the Racquette River. On the first pond was Dukett's Hiawatha Lodge. Turning left at the river, a sportsman could go upriver to Mother Johnson's Racquette Falls Lodge at the foot of the falls. After carrying around the falls, and going further upstream, one entered the fourteen miles of Long Lake where Uncle Palmer's, and Sabattis' lodges were located. Continuing toward the Fulton Chain were favorite spots like Cary's Rustic Lodge between Forked Lake and Racquette Lake. Another route was to go right at the Racquette River and down river to Moody's Mt. Morris House at the foot of Big Tupper Lake and McClure's Tupper Lake House at the other end. At the northern end of Upper Saranac was Hough's Prospect House at Saranac Inn (Murray, 1869, pp. 40–48; Donaldson, 1921, pp. 293–311; Correspondence, Janet Decker, Adirondack Room, Saranac Lake Public Library; see Map 6.1).

The availability of accommodations indicates that the few settlers in this region of the mountains were already entrepreneurs. They entertained city "sports" (as they were called locally) for hunting, fishing, and vacationing in the wilderness. And they accommodated those who exploited the region for its lumber, minerals, and ice.

Enthusiastic after their explorations, a variety of well-known authors published books and articles on their travels and adventures (Cadbury, 1989, p. 62). "All told of the beauties and health-giving qualities of the region, of its wealth of fish and game, and its possibilities for adventure" (Donaldson, 1921, p. 193). To illustrate the "health-giving qualities of the region," many told of invalids benefiting from the climate. One of the most popular books was *Adventures in the Wilderness,* published in 1869, and written by William Henry Harrison Murray, the pastor at Park Street Church in Boston, the center of evangelical Congregationalism in New England. He began regular vacations in 1866, usually camping on Racquette Lake (Cadbury, 1989, p. 62).

Murray's book became a best-seller because it was the first "how to do it" book, giving very practical information (Figure 6.1).

A tourist edition was published and "given free to those buying round trip tickets on the railroad from Boston to the Adirondacks" (Cadbury, 1989, p. 45). Published when he was in medical school, it is possible that Trudeau, E. H. Harriman, and the Livingstons had used the book for their earlier trips to the area.

To illustrate the health-giving qualities of the region, Murray wrote the following:

Another reason why I visit the Adirondacks, and urge others to do so, is because I deem the excursion eminently adapted to restore impaired health. Indeed, it is marvellous what benefit physically is often derived from a trip of a few weeks to these woods. To

Map 6.1

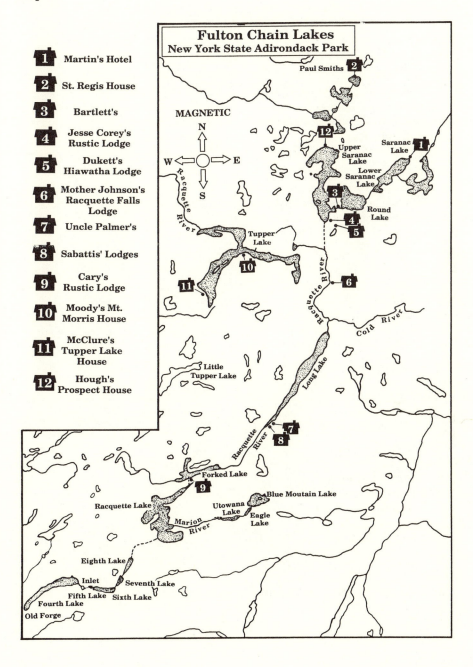

1	Martin's Hotel
2	St. Regis House
3	Bartlett's
4	Jesse Corey's Rustic Lodge
5	Dukett's Hiawatha Lodge
6	Mother Johnson's Racquette Falls Lodge
7	Uncle Palmer's
8	Sabattis' Lodges
9	Cary's Rustic Lodge
10	Moody's Mt. Morris House
11	McClure's Tupper Lake House
12	Hough's Prospect House

Fulton Chain Lakes
New York State Adirondack Park

Paul Smiths **2**

MAGNETIC
N
W ⟵ ⟶ E
S

Saranac Lake **1**

Upper Saranac Lake
Lower Saranac Lake

3

Round Lake
4
5

Racquette River

Tupper Lake
10

11

Racquette River

6

Cold River

Little Tupper Lake

Long Lake

7
8

Forked Lake
9

Blue Moutain Lake
Utowana Lake
Racquette Lake
Eagle Lake
Marion River

Eighth Lake
Inlet
Seventh Lake
Fifth Lake Sixth Lake
Fourth Lake
Old Forge

Figure 6.1
Table of Contents of *Adventures in the Wilderness* **by William H. H. Murray**

such as are afflicted with that dire parent of ills, dyspepsia, or have lurking in their system consumptive tendencies, I most earnestly recommend a month's experience among the pines. The air which you there inhale is such as can be found only in high mountainous regions, pure, rarefied, and bracing. The amount of venison steak a consumptive will consume after a week's residence in that appetizing atmosphere is a subject of daily and increasing wonder. I have known delicate ladies and fragile school-girls, to whom all food at home was distasteful and eating a pure matter of duty, average a gain of a pound per day for the round trip. This is no exaggeration, as some who will read these lines know. The spruce, hemlock, balsam, and pine, which largely compose this wilderness, yield upon the air, and especially at night, all their curative qualities. Many a night have I laid down upon my bed of balsam-boughs and been lulled to sleep by the murmur of waters and the low sighing melody of the pines, while the air was laden with the mingled perfume of cedar, of balsam and the water-lily. Not a few, far advanced in that dread disease, consumption, have found in this wilderness renewal of life and health. I recall a young man, the son of wealthy parents in New York, who lay dying in that great city, attended as he was by the best skill that money could secure. A friend calling upon him one day chanced to speak of the Adirondacks, and that many had found help from a trip to their region. From that moment he pined for the woods. He insisted on what his family called "his insane idea," that the mountain air and the aroma of the forest would cure him. It was his daily request and entreaty that he might go. At last his parents consented, the more readily because the physicians assured them that their son's recovery was impossible, and his death a mere matter of time. When he arrived at the point where he was to meet his guide he was too reduced to walk. The guide seeing his condition refused to take him into the woods, fearing, as he plainly expressed it, that he would "die on his hands." At last another guide was prevailed upon to serve him, not so much for the money, as he afterwards told me, but because he pitied the young man, and felt that "one so near death as he was should be gratified even in his whims."

The boat was half filled with cedar, pine, and balsam boughs, and the young man, carried in the arms of his guide from the house, was laid at full length upon them. The camp utensils were put at one end, the guide seated himself at the other, and the little boat passed with the living and the dying down the lake, and was lost to the group watching them amid the islands to the south. This was in early June. The first week the guide carried the young man on his back over all the portages, lifting him in and out of the boat as he might a child. But the healing properties of the balsam and pine, which were his bed by day and night, began to exert their power. Awake or asleep, he inhaled their fragrance. Their pungent and healing odors penetrated his diseased and irritated lungs. The second day out his cough was less sharp and painful. At the end of the first week he could walk by leaning on the paddle. The second week he needed no support. The third week the cough ceased entirely. From that time he improved with wonderful rapidity. He "went in" the first of June, carried in the arms of his guide. The second week of November he "came out" bronzed as an Indian, and as hearty. In five months he had gained sixty-five pounds of flesh, and flesh, too, "well packed on," as they say in the woods. Coming out he carried the boat over all portages; the very same over which a few months before the guide had carried him, and pulled as strong an oar as any amateur in the wilderness. His meeting with his family I leave the reader to imagine. The wilderness received him almost a corpse. It returned him to his home and the world as happy and healthy a man as ever bivouacked under its pines.

This, I am aware, is an extreme case, and, as such, may seem exaggerated; but it is not. I might instance many other cases which, if less startling, are equally corroborative of the general statement. There is one sitting near me, as I write, the color of whose cheek, and the clear brightness of whose eye, cause my heart to go out in ceaseless gratitude to the woods, amid which she found that health and strength of which they are the proof and sign. For five summers have we visited the wilderness. From four to seven weeks, each year, have we breathed the breath of the mountains; bathed in the waters which sleep at their base; and made our couch at night of moss and balsam-boughs, beneath whispering trees. I feel therefore, that I am able to speak from experience touching this matter; and I believe that, all things being considered, no portion of our country surpasses, if indeed equals, in health-giving qualities, the Adirondack Wilderness (Murray, 1869, pp. 11–15).

The parallels with Trudeau's experience are uncanny. Because consumption was considered to be fatal and physicians had no other remedies, change of climate held out some hope. Murray lectured extensively from 1870 to 1873, speaking "over five hundred times in the villages and cities of New England to nearly half a million people" (Cadbury, 1989, p. 53). Publicity about the region in the 1870s and 1880s, augmented by improved transportation to the mountains and entrepreneurial railroads, wilderness guides, and hotel owners, made the Adirondacks an attractive hunting, fishing, and vacationing area.

The mentality of New England was changing also.

The old puritan prejudice against play was becoming tempered by a growing realization of its benefits. Travel and outdoor pastimes, previously the privilege of a very small aristocracy, at least in New England, were coming to be viewed as a democratic right by more and more working people seeking to escape the confining pressures of industrial urbanization. Although resistance to the idea of recreation remained in some quarters, an increasingly large part of the public was both ready and willing to be convinced that recreation was a good thing (Cadbury, 1989, pp. 66–67).

In a sermon, Murray said, "Go anywhere where you can forget your cares and cast aside your burdens. . . . Let the old, old nurse, Nature, . . . take you to her bosom again; and you will return, to the city happier and healthier for the embrace" (Cadbury, 1989, pp. 66–68). The idea that nature could heal did not come just from homeopathic physicians, but from the personal testimonies of those fortunate enough to escape the smells, smoke, and filth of northeastern industrial cities. Faced with doing nothing and dying in a city, going into the woods, where many testified they had been healed, became an acceptable alternative. These personal testimonies may have led doctors like Loomis and Trudeau to go to the Adirondacks for their own health in the 1870s and 1880s. The general confidence that nature had healing properties may have been the reason that Loomis gave his 1879 speech. It was certainly the motive for Dr. Joseph Stickler to publish *The Adirondacks as a Health Resort* in 1886:

Several years before the publication of his book Dr. Stickler went to the mountains for a severe bronchitis, and found immediate and permanent relief. While traveling around he met so many invalids who had been helped by Adirondack air that their number impressed him. He decided that many more could be benefitted if the possibilities were made more widely known. In this altruistic spirit he wrote to a number of doctors and patients for testimonials of experience concerning the Adirondacks. The numerous replies are published in his book, and form an authoritative record of early health-seekers. Not all of them were tuberculous, but the majority were. Most of the experiences were prior to 1880; many of them prior to 1870. . . . The many scattered cases make an imposing number in the aggregate, and show clearly an instinctive tendency to gravitate toward these mountains, for tubercular relief, long before science had discovered the warrant for the impulse (Donaldson, 1921, pp. 266–67).

When Trudeau was deciding to set up the Sanitorium experiment the popular press, medical authorities, and the medical literature supported the idea. Nature, in general, and the Adirondacks, in particular, were places of healing. Stickler's book (1886) revealed that for twenty years before Trudeau opened the Adirondack Cottage Sanitarium a constant parade of well-to-do visitors traveled to the Adirondack region to improve their health. These were primarily business people, physicians, and clergy who could afford rustic lodgings and a guide or to build their own camp. Those whose work in factories, stores, and offices confined them to mill towns of the Northeast and cities like New York and Boston had little hope of enjoying similar benefits. If tuberculosis were to be treated, it was this level of society that had the greatest need and the greatest numbers, providing a fertile source of cases for Trudeau's sanitorium experiment. Other mountain sanitoria around the country benefitted as well (Clapesattle, 1984, p. 35).

Among those who came to Saranac Lake as wealthy patients was Mrs. C. M. Lea, the young wife of a Philadelphia publisher of medical books. Mrs. Lea, who stayed through the winter, was befriended by Lottie, and the families were close. Trudeau often discussed medical subjects with her husband, and Mr. Lea became one of the four original sanitarium trustees. Another patient was a businessman, Mr. D. W. Riddle, who was seriously ill but expressed great interest in Trudeau's ideas. After regaining his health, Riddle moved his family to the Adirondacks and took over "the practical problems of finances, building, and administration" and was treasurer of the sanitarium for thirty years. Trudeau had the unique skill of attracting talented people to his cause.

Loomis began to send patients to Dr. Trudeau. They boarded in local homes, and in the Berkeley Hotel after 1877, and were cared for by Trudeau. These were probably the twenty patients mentioned in Loomis's 1879 article. As Trudeau had more patients to attend, he began to take more interest in his profession. "Up to 1880 I did little but hunt and fish, but after that my interest began gradually to be divided equally between medicine and hunting. In the nineties I hunted only when I could get away from my work" (Trudeau, 1915, p. 137).

Also in 1879 Trudeau began to read medical journals. His health continued to improve. "I lost my cough almost entirely and gained weight, though my endurance to fatigue never became normal and any active exercise made me very short of breath" (Trudeau, 1915, p. 152).

About this time Trudeau discovered that he could raise funds quite success-fully. He realized this during their first winter (1875–76) in Saranac Lake. "I raised a subscription to subsidize the two-horse stage to Ausable Forks . . . to run daily instead of three times a week, and in this way we got mail regularly, except in the early spring when the roads were almost impassable and the stage ran somewhat irregularly" (Trudeau, 1915, p. 123).

In the fall of 1876 Trudeau began to raise money for a log chapel near Paul Smith's hotel where any clergyman guest might hold summer services. He appealed to the wealthy hotel guests as well as to his aunt, Mrs. Louis Livingston. The funds, materials, land, and furnishings were donated, and the chapel seating forty people was completed September 1877 with an invalid (tuberculosis patient) clergyman in charge for the summer. Trudeau com-mented: "This was the beginning of a lifetime of begging money from my friends, an occupation I have carried on unceasingly, and, thanks to the constancy of their friendship, rather successfully for forty years" (Trudeau, 1915, p. 127).

A similar campaign was led by Trudeau to build a Protestant Episcopal church in the village of Saranac Lake in 1878, and the Church of St. Luke the Beloved Physician was completed by the summer of 1879. Trudeau served as warden of the church vestry for the rest of his life (Trudeau, 1915, p. 151). Not only did these efforts give Dr. Trudeau confidence in his ability to raise funds, they also established his status in the local and wealthy summer communities. Also, he had the support of Dr. Alfred Loomis and was well connected to other prominent physicians who could provide a steady supply of patients.

In 1882, these capabilities were stirred by Trudeau's reading of an article in one of Luis Walton's old *English Practitioners*. He wrote:

The idea of building the Sanitarium originated on my reading . . . an account of a visit to Brehmer's Sanitarium in Silesia and a discussion of Brehmer's views as to the value of sanitorium treatment in pulmonary tuberculosis. Brehmer was the originator of the sanatorium method, the essence of which was rest, fresh air and a daily regulation by the physician of the patient's life and habits. Brehmer, however, had an idea that tuberculosis of the lungs was somewhat dependent on, or at least related to a small heart, and after the fever had fallen he attached more importance to graded climbing exercises for his patients to strengthening the heart.

Dettweiler, a patient and pupil of his . . . followed Brehmer's method, except that Dettweiler was an ardent advocate of complete rest, and he did not believe that a small heart had any special relation to pulmonary tuberculosis. I was much impressed with the articles . . . though I saw no reference to either Brehmer's or Dettweiler's work in my American journals. I became desirous of making a test of this new method in treating some of my tuberculous patients (Trudeau, 1915, p. 154).

The hopeful idea that tuberculosis could respond to total rest in the open air was accepted in Europe by the 1870s. Brehmer had established his sanitorium in 1854 in the Silesian Mountains and Dettweiler's sanitorium in the Taurus Mountains began in 1876. Here patients spent months resting on open-air balconies, breathing the "health-giving resinous aroma" of the pine forests. "Davos in the Swiss Alps became recognized as the best place to inhale pure air" (Taylor, 1986, p. 63). The European suggestions of Brehmer and Dettweiler fit very well with Trudeau's own personal experience. Brehmer, a botany student, suffered from tuberculosis and had gone to the Himalaya Mountains to do botanical studies and find a better climate to cure his disease. Returning home cured, he studied medicine and "presented a thesis on the subject 'Tuberculosis is Curable' " in 1854, the same year he established his sanitorium (Waksman, 1964, p. 63). Trudeau had not improved with exercising in Aiken, South Carolina, or in St. Paul, but he had improved when he went to the Adirondack Mountains and rested completely, exercising only when he felt well enough. "Daily regulation by the physician" gave Trudeau a role, which up to this point had not been defined.

Though Trudeau's wealthy patients could easily afford guides to care for them in rented cottages or at camps in the wilderness "there was absolutely no place for the working men and women who came here with short purses. It therefore occurred to me that a good piece of work could be done in helping these invalids, for whom my sympathy ever since my brother's death had always been keen, by building a few small cottages where they could be taken at a little less than cost and where the sanatorium method could be tried" (Trudeau, 1915, p. 155).

To try out a sanitorium experiment Trudeau needed a location and a source of willing patients. When he saw Dr. Alfred Loomis in the summer of 1882, Trudeau interested him in the experiment "where I could test Brehmer's and Dettweiler's rest, open-air and sanitorium methods . . . [on] some of the poor sick people in cities. He approved at once, and said he would be glad to send me such patients as they applied to him in the city, and that he would examine them free of charge. This he did to the day of his death in 1895, and gave the institution the support of his great name" (Trudeau, 1915, pp. 157–58).

Trudeau again solicited money from his wealthy friends and patients or their relatives. Because he vowed to contribute his own services to this experience, his pleas for funds had the tone of requesting money for missionary work among the urban poor who suffered from the fatal disease of tuberculosis. The initial solicitation of funds was signed by the trustees: Charles M. Lea, Daniel M. Riddle, and Edward L. Trudeau. It tells us what Trudeau had in mind.

The excellent results which have been obtained in the cure of the early stages of consumption and other pulmonary diseases, by residence in the Adirondacks, have led to this charity. There are hundreds of men and women who, could they at the proper time avail themselves of the advantages offered by that climate and proper medical treatment, would be entirely restored to health. But the expense of the step forbids it, opportunity for improvement passes, and soon they are beyond help.

There are charities which offer to the consumptive a shelter wherein he may pass the last days of his life, but none hold any hope of cure. . . .

It is to supply a refuge to such unfortunates that this charity is undertaken. . . .

Beginning by purchasing a good farm, there will be erected thereon a suitable central building sufficient to accommodate the matron and servants, and furnish kitchen, sitting-room and dining-room for the inmates, around which fifteen small cottages of the cheapest kind, each to accommodate two persons, will be built. . . . In this way the injurious effects of overcrowding patients in one sleeping-room will be avoided, as they will be entirely separated except at meal times. The farm should be able to support six to eight cows, and its other products would go far toward the maintenance of the patients. Much of the work of the farm will be done by patients themselves when able. . . . When patients are sufficiently recovered to be discharged, but require a longer residence in the climate, efforts will be made to find employment for them in the neighborhood. Physicians, trustees, treasurer, etc., have all offered their services without remuneration, the expenses for salaries will, therefore, be reduced to a minimum. As the men and women, whom it is proposed to cure have generally been subjected to the worst hygienic conditions, it may reasonably be expected that removal to such a climate as that of the ADIRONDACKS, with good food and proper medical treatment, results will be accomplished which are not usually obtained among patients accustomed to better sanitary surroundings (Board of Trustees Minutes, 1884).

This solicitation for "The Adirondack Cottages for the Cure of Pulmonary Diseases" appears to be patterned after many of the agrarian communal experiments that flourished in the century. The Shakers are a prominent example (Nordhoff, 1875). The idea of separate, clean cottages had been suggested by Florence Nïghtingale in the 1850s (Fleming, 1987, p. 85).

On a trip in the late winter and early spring of 1883 to New York, Trudeau raised over $3,000 to put up a small building. The Adirondack guides contributed sixteen acres of land costing $400.

He decided to separate patients in small cottages for nonmedical reasons, as he did not at that time believe tuberculosis was contagious.

I felt that aggregation should be avoided, and that segregation, such as could be secured by the cottage plan, would be preferable for many reasons. By adopting this plan an abundant supply of air could be secured for the patient, the visitation of constant close contact with many strangers could be avoided, and I knew it would be easier to get some of my patients to give a little cottage which would be their own individual gift, rather than a corresponding sum of money toward the erection of larger buildings (Trudeau, 1915, pp. 167–68).

Having experienced the crowded wards of Stranger's Hospital, Trudeau, who valued the solitude of the forest, fortuitously decided to segregate his patients in small cottages. He wrote: "When later the transmissibility of tuberculosis by the tubercle bacillus became generally accepted, I had reason to be thankful that I had from the first adopted the cottage plan" (Trudeau, 1915, p. 168). By midsummer 1884 part of a main building had been completed enough to move in the Norton family. Mr. Norton had been a small farmer and did the outside maintenance of the place, his wife and two daughters (18 and 15) did the cooking, housekeeping, and inside work. "Of course none of these people had ever heard of a sanitarium, or had the slightest idea of what it was intended to do, except to furnish board and lodging to a few invalids" (Trudeau, 1915, p. 169).

Dr. Loomis sent the first two patients in the late fall of 1884,

two sisters, both factory girls—one, Alice Hunt had pulmonary tuberculosis, and the other, Mary Hunt, had had Pott's disease and now showed slight evidences of pulmonary tuberculosis as well. Dr. Loomis had found someone willing to pay their expenses and had sent them up on this account, as nothing would have been done for them at their home, a crowded tenement. They were both in wretched health, poorly clad to stand the Adirondack winter cold, and were nearly dead with fatigue when they reached the Sanitarium after a forty-two mile drive from Ausable Forks. Mrs. Norton and her daughters took them right into the family circle, my wife got some warm clothes for them and I examined them and advised them to the best of my ability (Trudeau, 1915, p. 169).

At this point Trudeau did not have a systematically thought out theory about how to treat tuberculosis. He must have been sympathetic to Brehmer's and Dettweiler's methods, as they corresponded to his own experience. Because he had improved while resting and living an outdoor life in the mountains, he knew that rest and fresh air were important. He had learned this from the Adirondack guides—Paul Smith, Warren Flanders, Fred Martin, and others. As most consumptives were weak and thin, it seemed logical to follow Alonzo Clark's general treatment, which included the best food and clean air. Rigid regimens did not exist at the beginning.

What Trudeau called the "outdoor life cure" for tuberculosis used the homeopathic idea of rest and nourishment to help the body fight and repel the disease. He followed Alonzo Clark's advice almost literally—good food, walking in the open air, active friction on the skin, and cod-liver oil. What perhaps was more important, for the first time in the history of this major killer disease there was acceptance by some in the medical establishment that this "cure" was effective. As all families, rich and poor, had experienced consumption, which accounted for about one in seven deaths and had been assumed fatal, a certified "cure" attracted great medical and lay attention. That it was partly imported from Europe and practiced by a tall cosmopolitan gentleman with a slight French accent who had recovered from it himself gave it additional reputation in the eyes of many, especially the patients. These factors may have had considerable healing influence for those who believed them.

Learning about the Tubercle Bacillus

In the fall of 1885 Trudeau added another room (8 by 12 feet) to his house for a laboratory and began investigations that excited him the rest of his life. After learning to stain and identify the tubercle bacillus, he wanted to culture it outside the human body and produce the disease in laboratory animals, as Koch had done. The technique for doing this required growing the bacillus on solidified blood.

I bought a small sheep for three dollars and a half, and from the sacrifice of this animal I procured the required amount of blood, which thanks to the pure air and the snow on the ground, remained tolerably free from contamination and was transferred at once to the ice box to coagulate. I am afraid my associates at the laboratory today would hardly consider the technique I then employed up to date, but after many accidents I succeeded in getting some fair plants of blood serum in tubes.

I made plants on this blood serum from a tuberculous gland removed from one of my inoculated guinea pigs, and put all the tubes in my home-made thermostat. . . . Many of the tubes turned out at once to be contaminated, and a variety of growths appeared on them; but after ten days I still had four tubes free from contamination and these looked much as when I first put them in the incubator. On the eighteenth day I thought I detected a little growth in the corner of one of these. With every precaution against contamination, with my platinum spade I removed a little of the suspected growth and rubbed it on a couple of clean slides, dried it, and stained it. My first intimation of success was when one or two large masses on the slide refused to decolorize when treated with the acid. I washed the slide, put it under the microscope, and to my intense joy I saw nothing but well-stained culture masses and a few detached tubercle bacilli. I at once planted some fresh tubes from the one I had examined, and I knew now I had pure cultures to work with. This little scum on the serum was consumption in a tangible form. With it I could inoculate animals and try experiments to destroy the germ (Trudeau, 1915, pp. 202–203).

Despite the crudeness of his methods and facilities, Trudeau obtained living tubercle bacilli. Proud of his success he sent a tube to Dr. Welch at Hopkins and to his mentor at Columbia, Dr. Prudden, "as I knew he would be glad to show the students this recently discovered germ which kills one in seven of the human race" (Trudeau, 1915, p. 203).

Another glimpse at conditions in early days comes from Trudeau's efforts to keep laboratory animals. Rabbits he could keep alive with ease, but guinea pigs would die from the cold on winter evenings when the inside temperature of the house often went below freezing. "It became evident that I should have to keep my guinea pigs, as I did my potatoes, below ground. I had a big hole dug in my yard. . . . I put a kerosene lamp in this little cellar to heat it, and kept my guinea pigs in boxes on wooden shelves in this place. This, though most inconvenient when the animals had to be handled or treated, turned out to answer fairly well" (Trudeau, 1915, p. 204).

WAS TUBERCULOSIS A CONTAGIOUS DISEASE?

In order to understand how revolutionary Trudeau's work was in 1885 we have to look at the beliefs of physicians about this time. They did not accept the existence of germs and therefore could not agree that tuberculosis was contagious. In 1883, Dr. Shrady published the results of a survey of British physicians from the *British Medical Journal*. With 1,078 physicians responding, only 261 (24%) "affirmed the proposition that phthisis may be communicated." Despite these results Shrady opined, "The facts thus elicited show that a small proportion, probably less than five percent, of general practitioners have met with evidence which leads them to believe that consumption is contagious" (*Medical Record,* vol. 24, December 8, 1883, p. 629). In January 1885 he reported a similar survey of 680 Italian physicians in which only "59, or 8.6 per cent, believed in contagion" (*Medical Record,* vol. 27, January 17, 1885, p. 75). Shrady himself did not appear to accept the idea of contagion. At the meeting of the American Medical Association in the spring of 1884, physicians debated the contagiousness of consumption. A paper was read by Dr. Henry F. Formad of Philadelphia in which he reviewed the evidence and concluded "that tuberculosis was not a contagious disorder." In the following acrimonious discussion some physicians supported Formad, including Dr. G. Traill Green and Dr. William Pepper. But there was a longer list of physicians who went on public record to disagree, saying they felt tuberculosis was contagious—Dr. Austin Flint, Sr., Dr. George Sternberg, Dr. James Tyson, Dr. E. G. Janeway, and Dr. E. O. Shakespeare (*Medical Record,* vol. 25, May 10, 1884, pp. 527–28). All of those disagreeing were acquaintances of Edward Trudeau, and several became members of the renegade Association of American Physicians formed in 1886.

The idea that tuberculosis was caused by a germ created major difficulties for most physicians who had been taught to believe that consumption was hereditary—that people inherited weak dispositions or predispositions toward the disease. Once it was suggested that the tubercle bacillus was always present in cases of tuberculosis and therefore was very likely causal, the next question had to do with why one person became infected and others, though equally exposed, resisted the bacilli's invasion. Here again, the question of hereditary predisposition arose. Were some disposed by heredity to have greater susceptibility, or was it a question of the person's general health?

For those who had been trained to think of heredity, susceptibility was still a possibility. But others asked what conditions produced a "soil" receptive to the growth of the bacillus "seed." They concluded that in many cases the seed grew in a soil made susceptible by malnutrition, poor working conditions, and inadequate housing. Some pointed out the obvious class differences in tuberculosis, comparing the well-nourished with the poorly nourished (*Medical Record,* vol. 29, June 5, 1886, p. 688). Edward Trudeau was beginning to accept the germ theory, believed in contagion, and understood that those with poor nutrition who came from poor environments were more susceptible to the bacillus. Though the majority of physicians were not convinced by Koch's paper (or had not read translations of it), Trudeau became very interested and set about to convince himself and others.

In the summer of 1885 his physician and source of referrals, Alfred Loomis, was back for his annual vacation in the Adirondacks. Loomis did not believe in germs and was unwilling to accept microscopic evidence for tuberculosis. Trudeau wrote:

A young college student had come . . . while on his vacation to consult Dr. Loomis for a slight but persistent cough and some loss of weight and strength. But Dr. Loomis was away in camp and somehow the young man asked me to prescribe for his cough. On examination of the chest I could find nothing positive, but I was so keen about my newly acquired knowledge in staining the tubercle bacillus that I subjected every patient who coughed to this test. To my astonishment I found the germ present in the expectoration, and told the patient he had tuberculosis and should not return to college in the fall, but go West and lead an outdoor life for a time [Trudeau had adopted Alonzo Clark's suggestion]. Naturally his family was much alarmed, for he was a big, strong man and they had no idea there would be anything serious the matter with him. He awaited Dr. Loomis' return at Paul Smith's in order to get his opinion. Dr. Loomis, who of course attached no special importance to the presence of the bacillus, examined him thoroughly. He could find nothing definite the matter with his lungs and said he could see no reason why the young man should not continue his college course. . . . Four months later one of my patients at Saranac Lake told me he had just heard that this young man had had a serious hemorrhage in the class-room, and had been sent at once to Colorado (Trudeau, 1915, pp. 183–84).

Presumably Loomis heard about this case and was impressed. When he published the second edition of the *Practice of Medicine* in 1890, he sent a copy to Trudeau with the suggestion that he read the chapter on tuberculosis. Finally, Loomis had become convinced that germs did indeed exist.

Local physicians were just as skeptical as Loomis. The following story illustrates Trudeau's approach to his colleagues:

I had many opportunities to convince the unbelieving. Dr. D'Arignon had practiced medicine and surgery at Ausable Forks and was called upon in consultation and to operate all over the mountains. He was a shrewed, resourceful and skillful surgeon, and thoroughly interested in his profession. On one of his visits to Saranac Lake he called on me and found me in the little laboratory. He asked me about "the germs," in which he had as yet little faith; but he said "Will you take the trouble to convince me?" [Perhaps by 1885 he had heard of Joseph Lister's success at killing bacteria in surgical wounds.] I asked him what test he required, and he said, "I will send you five numbered samples and if you can tell me which ones came from tuberculosis cases and which ones did not, I will believe it all." I agreed, and he left, evidently thinking he had me cornered.

The samples came, with only a number on each one, and I reported on them at once. Three contained bacilli and I wrote him the result and gave him the numbers. A more convinced and enthusiastic man than he was when he made his next visit I never saw. He had lost his contempt for "germs," and the little ironical smile he wore on his last visit as he looked at my culture tubes had disappeared. After that when he had doubtful cases he often sent me samples for examination, and the results left his new faith unshaken (Trudeau, 1915, pp. 185–86).

D'Arignon had tried an experiment, and Trudeau had convinced him. But these trials went on for several years.

As late as 1890, a young Columbia College rowing man came to Paul Smith's for a troublesome cough he could not throw off, and I detected the bacillus on the first examination and told him he had tuberculosis. He smiled and said I must be mistaken, for he had rowed a good race on the crew that spring, and had just been insured by two of the best insurance companies in New York for a large sum. I made another examination, found the germ and reiterated my opinion. This brought a letter from one of the insurance companies asking me on what I based my diagnosis. I answered that the symptoms were very suspicious, but that the presence of the bacillus, in my mind, was irrefutable evidence of the presence of a tuberculous process as their cause. An interval followed, then a very nice note came from the insurance company asking me whether, if they sent up one of their doctors, I would show him my method of detecting the bacillus and making such a diagnosis. The doctor arrived. I showed him how to find the bacillus and he departed the next day. Within a couple of days I received a nice note of thanks from the insurance company and a check for one hundred dollars. The patient died several years later of tuberculosis (Trudeau, 1915, pp. 184–85).

It took a long time for American physicians to accept germs and the evidence of bacteriology. Presumably the insurance company physician could have learned the same technique from Dr. Prudden or Dr. Hodenpyl in New York City. Perhaps it was safer to admit ignorance to someone outside the city, though by 1890 Trudeau was developing a reputation as one of the most knowledgeable about tuberculosis in this country.

These incidents were evidence that did much to convince the skeptical medical profession that the tubercle bacillus existed and could be reliably identified and used in diagnosis. By participating in these experiments with his colleagues, Trudeau developed a reputation as a medical scientist, bringing recognition and prestige to his sanitarium and laboratory. Physicians sent more patients to Saranac Lake and came themselves when symptoms developed. While these experiments convinced his colleagues that Trudeau was an authority on tuberculosis, he was pursuing another course. Weakened by his own disease, Trudeau could still enjoy the comradeship and accomplishment of a good hunt with medical colleagues in his laboratory.

Now that the source of the disease was in his hands, Trudeau could try a new approach. If the bacillus could be cultured, it could be destroyed. As Lister used carbolic acid on surgical wounds, Trudeau searched for a substance that would kill the tubercle bacillus. In 1885, this kind of thinking was not accepted by American physicians.

In April 1883, T. Mitchell Prudden had published a study raising a question about the universality of Koch's findings (*Medical Record,* vol. 23, April 14, 1883, pp. 397–400). Another paper by Prudden in June agreed that microscopic sputum examination

must become a part of the professional furnishing of every expert diagnostician, whether the bacilli stand in a causative relation to tuberculosis or not (p. 645).

It is very essential that it be clearly understood that its occurrence in sputum and other excreta in tuberculosis, however constant or practically valuable as a means of diagnosis, is not in itself a proof of the parasitic origin of the disease, nor does the search for it commit the observer in the least to the germ theory. For as far as all this goes, it may be merely a harmless concomitant of tuberculosis and nothing more. When once it is proven beyond reasonable doubt to be one of the causes or the sole cause of tuberculosis in man, then will arise questions in prophylaxis and therapeutics second in importance to none which can engage the attention of medical men (*Medical Record,* vol. 23, June 16, 1883, p. 648).

George Sternberg, a physician in the U.S. Army posted in rural Kansas, presented a paper to the Biology Section of the American Association for the Advancement of Science. He stated "that he had repeated Koch's inoculation experiments and was able to confirm him as to the infectious nature of tuberculosis." (*Medical Record,* vol. 26, September 20, 1884, p. 317).

Finally in September 1885, Shrady's editorial in the *Medical Record* (vol. 28, September 19, 1885, pp. 322–23) argued that "the importance of the bacillus tuberculosis in the diagnostic study of phthisis is now universally admitted." It is likely that these papers challenged Trudeau to present evidence supporting Koch.

In his first scientific paper, "An Experimental Research Upon the Infectiousness of Non-bacillary Phthisis," Trudeau (1885) investigated "whether non-bacillary phthisical sputum possesses any infectious qualities" (p. 361). After Trudeau had examined the sputum of twenty-nine people with phthisis, all of whom had bacilli, the thirtieth patient's sputum did not produce the tubercle bacillus. Repeated examinations for two months could not detect bacilli in this woman's sputum. Her case history was given to illustrate that she had all the symptoms of tuberculosis. From these efforts Trudeau concluded that "non-bacillary phthisis is a comparatively rare disease" (p. 364).

Following the work of Prudden and Sternberg, Trudeau then performed this experiment on twelve full-grown rabbits:

Four were inoculated with bacillary sputum from a patient with chronic phthisis; four with the expectoration of a healthy person attacked with acute bronchitis; while the remaining four were injected with non-bacillary phthisical sputum from the case selected. . . . The animals were then kept entirely separate under the best possible conditions with respect to food, light, and air.

In the animals injected with bacillary sputum, the results were much the same as found by other observers. . . . In every case at the point of inoculation . . . tubercle bacilli were easily demonstrated. . . .

In the four rabbits injected with the sputum of simple bronchitis . . . the most thorough search failed to reveal any bacilli. . . .

In all the four rabbits injected with non-bacillary phthisical expectoration, slight, purely localized inflammatory changes resulted, in none of which tubercles or the characteristic bacilli could be detected.

From these results, Trudeau concluded:

that possibly the patient from whom the sputum was obtained was not suffering from phthisical disease at all; if so, we must acknowledge our inability to diagnosticate the disease, for the case presented all the rational and physical signs of pulmonary tuberculosis, and until the sputum was examined nothing led to any suspicion that it differed in any way from the many others under observation. . . .

Such evidence must tend to strengthen the sinister claims of Koch's bacillus, and another failure recorded in an attempt to produce tuberculosis without its agency (Trudeau, 1885, pp. 361–65).

This paper provided evidence to support Koch's findings. With it, Trudeau lined up on the side of the new medical science that accepted what the bacteriologists were saying about these unique microorganisms called tubercle bacilli or germs or parasites or viruses. About the name there was little agreement. The importance of the bacillus in the diagnosis of tuberculosis had been accepted. Even Dr. Hodenpyl, Prudden's assistant at Physicians and Surgeons, published "A case of acute general tuberculosis diagnosticated during life by the presence of tubercle bacilli in the sputum" (*Medical Record,* vol. 28, November 21, 1885). Dr. Hodenpyl became a patient at the sanitarium in 1897.

Once the bacillus was accepted as the causal agent for tuberculosis, medical thinking began to shift. No longer was heredity necessary to account for the existence of tuberculosis in families, and those who believed it was contagious finally began to represent the majority (Waksman, 1964, pp. 50–54). Dr. Henry Didama from Onondaga County gave a paper at the second annual meeting of the New York State Medical Association entitled "Tubercular Consumption—Is It Ever Inherited?" He argued that children become phthisical because "they are living in an atmosphere of the disease and thus are more exposed than other children." He recommended isolating the child from the phthisical parent (*Medical Record,* vol. 28, November 21, 1885, p. 577). Physicians began to change from "heredity" to "contagion" as the means by which tuberculosis was transmitted. Thus, the disease fit into a model physicians already possessed for a disease like syphilis. (Contagion had been suggested earlier, in 1880, by Conheim and Whittaker, as noted in chapter 5.) Once this familial contagion was understood, physicians began to recognize it in their practices and report examples. Earlier in the century, examples of whole families succumbing to tuberculosis had certified that tuberculosis was hereditary. Now that germs and the mechanism of infection had been discovered, the same examples indicated that it was contagious.

EXAMPLES OF CONTAGION

An original article by James King Crook reported on fifty-nine cases of pulmonary consumption collected between June and September of 1885. After noting that most of the patients were in their twenties, employed in indoor occupations, and born in America, the author concluded, "The foregoing data constituted our chief reasons for regarding pulmonary consumption as an infectious or contagious disease" (*Medical Record,* vol. 29, March 13 and 20, 1886, p. 323).

Case studies of individuals caring for phthisical patients appeared. A girl looking after a dying tubercular patient cut her finger on a piece of broken glass from the patient's cuspidor. In two weeks she was infected. Compresses of carbolic acid abated the infection, but the girl was found to be tubercular (*American Journal of the Medical Sciences,* vol. 89, April 1885, pp. 571–72).

Shrady mentioned another survey, this one among French physicians. Of the 123 who responded, fifty-seven or 46 percent said they believed in contagion. The proportion of physicians accepting contagion was increasing, but acceptance by civil authorities would take much longer. Class differences were mentioned, also. "It is roughly estimated to be one in ten among the well-fed classes, among the poor classes it is much greater" (*Medical Record,* vol. 29, June 5, 1886, p. 668). Another study reported 123 autopsies of infants at the pathological institute of Kiel University. Shrady summarized: "Basing his opinion on the fact that no tuberculosis was found post-mortem in children under nine weeks of age, Dr. Schwer concludes that tuberculosis is never a congenital or connate [acquired at birth] disease." Unwilling to give up on heredity completely, Shrady made the following methodological point. "Dr. Schwer's view that tuberculosis is never congenital is not borne out either by his own statistics or those of others. It is only probable, and not certain, that the infants who died of tuberculosis at the age of nine weeks were not born with the disease" (*Medical Record,* vol. 29, June 19, 1886, p. 713).

Trudeau entered this debate with a brief case report of a twenty-four-year-old woman who became a "child's nurse" to one of his patients suffering from "advanced pulmonary phthisis with progressing excavation":

Five months later, in March 1886, I was asked to see her, as she had taken cold, and found her suffering from the usual symptoms of a moderate bronchitis. Two weeks later, being informed that she was still coughing, I examined her more carefully: her temperature was 100.75 degrees, pulse 90, skin moist, and tongue clean. In the chest nothing beyond marked feebleness of vesicular murmur at left apex and some scattered coarse rales in both lungs observed. As I was then making sputum examinations, it occurred to me to obtain a sample of the expectoration for study. To my astonishment, a few tubercle bacilli were detected and subsequent examination showed them in great numbers. A diagnosis of phthisis with its accompanying unfavorable prognosis was given. . . . When heard from again in September, she was failing rapidly and unable to be moved.

Trudeau concluded, "Deficient as any evidence of direct contagion in phthisis must always be, it must be conceded that many facts in the foregoing case seem to point to more than mere coincidence. The girl had always been healthy, there was no phthisis in her family, she was in a good climate and under excellent hygienic conditions when after less than five months of exposure the first symptoms of the phthisical process made their appearance and progressed uninterruptedly" (Trudeau, 1886, p. 464). With this case study, Trudeau provided evidence that tuberculosis was contagious and that the bacillus was the agent.

CLIMATE AND ITS RELATION TO TUBERCULOSIS

Another line of research in the medical literature concerned the question of climate. We have seen how various centers like Aiken, Asheville, and St. Paul were publicized by physicians. Evidence was presented to support Austin Flint's argument that tuberculosis was "self-limiting," that some people recovered spontaneously. Shrady reported on a paper presented to the British Medical Association by Dr. C. R. Drysdale, who concluded that because people recover from tuberculosis "under the most varied circumstances . . . phthisis is curable in a variety of circumstances too numerous to mention. . . . both theory and experience had shown that the pure air of high mountain districts and of the ocean, both of which localities were free from the impurities existing in inland places and low levels, were the climates, par excellence, for the cure of tuberculosis" (*Medical Record,* vol. 30, August 28, 1886, p. 246). Other papers stressed high altitudes (*Medical Record,* vol. 30, December 25, 1886, p. 708; vol. 31, January 15, 1887, p. 70; May 7, 1887, p. 527; May 14, 1887; and *Medical News,* vol. 51, July 23, 1887, pp. 88–91). Trudeau was interested in these issues, having become a member of the American Climatological Association in 1884, nominated by its president, Alfred Loomis.

In the spring of 1887 Trudeau gave a paper before the association that became a classic for Trudeau's followers (Trudeau, 1887a). In the first paragraph he revealed the tension in the medical profession. "The older clinical medicine on one side points to unhygienic surroundings, malnutrition, struma, defect of anatomical structure, and heredity as the main causes of tubercular disease, while experimental research brings evidence not easily to be thrust aside to support its claim to have discovered in the bacillus tuberculosis the virus which is essential to the production of this fatal class of maladies" (p. 131). Reviewing previous studies, Trudeau argued they established "the fact that environment is a most potent factor in the causation of tuberculosis." He then carried out an experiment to study the effects of environment on the progress of tubercular infection, using fifteen rabbits.

Experiment No. 1. Five rabbits were inoculated in the right lung and in the left side of the neck with five minims of sterilized water in which was suspended a sufficient quantity of a pure culture (third generation) of the tubercle bacillus to render the liquid quite perceptibly turbid. The needle of the Koch's inoculating syringe was inserted subcutaneously on the left side of the neck and in the third intercostal space to a depth of thirty millimeters on the right side. These animals were then confined in a small box and put in a dark cellar. They were thus deprived of light, fresh air, and exercise, and were also stinted in the quantity of food given them while being themselves artificially infected with the tubercle bacillus.

Experiment No. 2. Five healthy rabbits were placed under the following conditions: A fresh hole about ten feet deep was dug in the middle of a field, and the animals having been confined in a small box with high sides but no top, were lowered to the bottom of this pit, the mouth of which was then covered with boards and fresh earth. Through this covering a small trap door was cut which was only opened long enough each day to allow of the food consisting of a small potato to each rabbit, being thrown to the animals. So damp was the ground at the bottom of this pit that the box in which the rabbits were confined was constantly wet. Thus these animals were deprived of light, fresh air, and exercise, furnished with but a scanty supply of food while breathing a chill and damp atmosphere, though free from disease themselves and removed as far as possible from any accidental source of bacterial infection.

Experiment No. 3. Five rabbits having been inoculated in precisely the same manner as the animals in the first experiment were at once turned loose on a small island in June 1886. It would be difficult to imagine conditions better suited to stimulate the vitality of these animals to the highest point than were here provided. They lived all the time in the sunshine and fresh air, and soon acquired the habit of constant motion so common in wild animals. The grass and green shrubs on the island afforded all the fresh food necessary and, in addition, they were daily provided with an abundant supply of vegetables. Thus, while artificially infected themselves they were placed in the midst of conditions well adapted to stimulate their vital powers to the highest point attainable.

The results of these experiments were very interesting.

Experiment No. 1. Four of the inoculated rabbits confined in the cellar died within three months; in all of them the injected lung was extensively diseased; the other lung and the bronchial glands being also more or less involved and tubercles in various stages, but sufficiently advanced to be macroscopical, were found in the pleura, peritoneum, spleen, and liver; from these lesions pure cultures of tubercle bacilli were obtained. The fifth rabbit survived and was killed four months after injection; at the autopsy the right lung was found solidified and shrivelled, the upper portion being almost entirely destroyed, while a bronchial gland as large as a hazelnut, filled with creamy pus, occupied the right chest; tubercles, which in many places had become cheesy, studded the upper portion of the left lung. The other organs were healthy.

Experiment No. 2. The five uninoculated and healthy rabbits placed in the damp pit were all living at the end of four months. They were emaciated, and their coats were rough, but they still seemed about as active as at the beginning of the experiment. They were all killed within a few days of each other, but a careful examination of their organs revealed nothing abnormal in any of them.

Experiment No. 3. One of the five rabbits which were allowed to run at large died just one month after inoculation. The lower portion of the lung was solidified. The bronchial glands enlarged, as well as the axillary glands on the left side, and a few tubercles were made out in the spleen. The left lung and all the other organs were sound. The four other rabbits remained apparently in perfect health, and so active had they become that two of them could only be captured with the aid of a gun. All four animals were killed at the beginning of November, or four months after inoculation. They were loaded with adipose tissue, and their flesh was so firm and red as to be in striking contrast to the blanched and flabby muscles of the other rabbits previously examined. All the organs were healthy and even the points of inoculation could not be made out.

Trudeau's interpretation of these results is very interesting. First he said, "The evidence afforded by these experiments confirms the view that the production of tuberculosis is a most complex problem and one in which many elements besides the bacillus enter. How surely and rapidly this microbe accomplishes its work when the normal resisting power of the system is for any cause lowered, is well shown by the manner in which the first lot of animals succumbed. Localized tuberculosis was in every instance but one quickly followed by general systemic infection and death."

He added a methodological note: "That animals kept in most laboratories are frequently confined under conditions of air, light, and overcrowding, which may materially influence the results of investigations in a disease of the nature of tuberculosis, can hardly be denied and should be kept in view."

Commenting on the second experiment, Trudeau said: "The results obtained seem to indicate that unfavorable environment and the consequent malnutrition which invariably follows existence amidst unhygienic surroundings are not sufficient of themselves to cause tuberculosis." This outcome was evidence that the bacillus had to be present for the disease to develop under these poor conditions.

Regarding the third experiment, Trudeau wrote: "The fate of the animals allowed to run wild is most instructive, inasmuch as it seems to indicate that in a great majority of instances resistance to the invasion of so deadly a germ as the tubercle bacillus is possible in the artificially produced disease, provided the vital and nutritive processes of the animal are stimulated to the highest possible state of activity." Trudeau cautioned the reader to remember that in the animals "the tuberculosis was an artificial one, produced in previously sound animals, and not the culmination, as in the spontaneous disease in man and animals, of many debilitating causes, acting often through long periods of time, and impairing the resisting power of the system to such a degree as to allow of spontaneous infection."

Nevertheless, Trudeau felt these results raised an important question. "If, therefore, environment is so potent a factor in determining bacterial infection, are its effects on the future course of the malady when it has occurred to be disregarded? How potent may be its influence is demonstrated by the widely differing results obtained in the inoculated rabbits allowed to run wild, and those confined amidst unhygienic surroundings."

While the environment is important, it is only one factor. Trudeau placed his emphasis upon the "resisting power of the individual which may be computed as the sum total of all the conditions which affect individual vitality through heredity and environment." Trudeau then tied these findings into the new "phagocytosis hypothesis," which had been presented by Metchnikoff in 1883, as the first theory of immunity and the beginning of immunology. "Bacteriology already points to the cell as an active factor in resisting the progress of bacterial invasion. Metchnikoff saw the lymph cells of the frog englobe and destroy anthrax bacilli." Trudeau indicated that he was aware of the work of Pasteur and Koch on anthrax in 1876–77. "As the pathogenic qualities of infectious germs may in many instances be abrogated or diminished at will, as in the preliminary manipulation of bacteria used in vaccinations, by placing them under peculiar conditions of environment which rob them of their virulence, or modify it, so may the resisting power of their natural enemies, the cells of the body, be diminished or increased by the same means."

The conclusion of this research was that

All measures which tend to increase the vitality of the body cells have been found to be precisely those which are most effectual in combating tuberculosis. Though environment may bear but the relation of a predisposing cause to microbic infection, it is, nevertheless, a potent factor in determining the future type, and even the final results of the disease, and that if we may not underestimate the pathogenic properties of the bacillus, the effect of extremes of environment on the resisting power of the cells of the body is an element in this complex problem which should not be ignored (Trudeau, 1887a, pp. 131–36).

The paper was first presented at the June 1887 meeting of the American Climatological Association, to which Trudeau had just been elected. Trudeau told this story about that experience.

It was the beginning of June, and terribly hot when we reached Baltimore that evening. I hardly slept at all that night. I don't think this was entirely due to the heat, however, as I was beginning to dread the idea of speaking in public before a large audience of doctors, and I am sure this kept me awake. The next day it was just as hot and I could eat no breakfast. I went to the meeting and found a large hall packed with medical men. I sat next to Dr. Loomis and listened to papers on the program, but it seemed a long session and the dread of having to speak before such an audience increased. [Trudeau was 39 years old.]

It was almost time for my paper when I began to feel dizzy and faint. I leaned over to Dr. Loomis and said, "Doctor I feel badly." He turned around and looked at me and said, "Get up and go out." I tried to, but just before I got to the door darkness overtook me and I fainted. The next thing I remember I was lying on the floor in the hall. . . . Dr. Loomis was leaning over me and saying, "Where is your paper?" I gave it to him, and then lay there in a sort of half-conscious state listening to Dr. Loomis's strong voice as he read my paper. Then came loud applause, and soon Dr. Loomis came back and handed me the paper and said, "That was a good paper." Other men crowded around me and shook hands with me, and spoke of the paper and hoped I was feeling all right again. I got on my feet and walked out into the street while somebody held my arm, and I soon began to feel much better. . . . I was thoroughly ashamed of myself, but there was no help for what had happened, and I tried to lay my fainting entirely to the excessive heat (Trudeau, 1915, pp. 207–208).

At this stage of his knowledge, Trudeau felt that this experiment explained what had happened in his own case and others he had observed healing in the woods. Climate could be a potent force in increasing the vitality of the individual so that the bacillus could be resisted. Science had already disclosed that tuberculosis was self-limiting, that thousands of people had successfully formed tubercles on their lungs that "englobed" the bacilli and prevented spread of the disease. How to encourage this process and modify the virulence of the bacillus became his goal. In Trudeau's experience a well-fed life of rest in the woods helped him. This "experimental research" provided "scientific" evidence that sanitorium care in the mountains could effectively treat tuberculosis. Although this experimental design would be unacceptable to today's scientists, in the 1880s the word "experiment" carried profound significance for physicians. It convinced Trudeau and his colleagues that sanitorium treatment was effective. By demonstrating that the poor environment of many in the lower classes contributed to the contagiousness of the disease, Trudeau aligned himself with the hygiene movement, which had become prominent in America after successfully preventing the spread of cholera in 1865.

At these meetings Trudeau met other people with similar sympathies such as William Osler and William H. Welch, men who were building the medical school at Johns Hopkins University. Osler, who was respected as a great clinician and teacher, mentioned the Adirondack Cottage Sanitarium in the first edition, in 1893, of his *Practice of Medicine*. [The 1913 edition contains chapters by Trudeau's colleagues Baldwin, chapter 4, and Brown, chapter 6.] Trudeau felt that it was Osler's influence that got him elected as the first president of the National Association for the Study and Prevention of Tuberculosis in 1905.

8

Attempts to Destroy the Bacillus

Although the environment might stimulate the body to resist the bacilli, more active efforts were being made to destroy them by other means. After Lister's visit to the United States the debate over his methods (see chapter 5) lasted several years. But it convinced surgeons that germs existed and that they could be destroyed on surgical sites. If carbolic and phenic acid sprays could kill bacteria on a surgical site, perhaps the tubercle bacillus could be killed by similar means.

Several disinfectants had been suggested, with carbolic acid being the most reliable and economical (*American Journal of Medical Sciences,* vol. 88, July 1884, p. 193, and October 1884, pp. 561–64). The contents of rooms and the clothes of those who had died from phthisis were to be disinfected. Numerous testimonials were given by physicians for their favorite disinfectants. The methods for applying these chemicals recall the "heroic" heritage of medicine from earlier periods. Some were to be inhaled:

- acetic ether (*Medical News,* vol. 41, July 15, 1882, p. 65)
- 5% solution of benzoate of soda in the form of a spray (*Medical News,* vol. 41, August 12, 1882, p. 181)
- iodoform (*Medical News,* vol. 43, July 14, 1883, p. 38)
- creosote, eucalyptol, carbolic acid, naphthols, bichloride of mercury (*Medical News,* vol. 45, October 25, 1884, p. 460)
- menthol (*Medical News,* vol. 50, July 4, 1887, p. 626)
- burning sulphur (*Medical Record,* vol. 23, February 17, 1883, p. 195; vol. 26, August 16, 1884, p. 194)

- oxygen and corrosive sublimate (*Medical Record,* vol. 25, January 5, 1884, p. 4)

- 20 drops of a mixture of equal parts creosote and chloroform dropped upon a sponge (*Medical Record,* vol. 24, October 13, 1883, p. 419)

- fluoric acid sprayed into a room (*Medical Record,* vol. 30, November 6, 1886, p. 519)

- compressed air laden with finely powdered and carefully dried Borax (*Medical News,* vol. 51, November 5, 1887, p. 542)

Other agents were to be mixed with the bacillus to kill it. Two British researchers studied the "action of various chemical reagents on the vitality of the bacillus tubercle" and published the following list in order of increasing effectiveness.

- lactic acid, camphoric acid (a saturated solution), camphor (a saturated alcoholic solution), bromide of ethyl, naphthol B, turpentine, chloride of palladium, creosote, naphthol Alpha, phenic acid, and bichloride of mercury (*Medical News,* vol. 47, November 21, 1885, p. 572)

Other researchers argued for:

- sulphurous acid (*Medical Record,* vol. 23, March 10, 1883, p. 278)

- steam (*American Journal of the Medical Sciences,* vol. 88, July 1884, p. 193)

Another method was injection of antiseptics directly into the diseased lung, using "dilute solutions of liq. iodinic comp., . . . [also] dilute solution of carbolic acid, and dilute Lugol's solution" (*Medical Record,* vol. 27, January 10, 1885, p. 31). Success with these injections was reported a year later by a practicing physician using intrapulmonary injections of carbolized iodine (*Medical Record,* vol. 30, November 13, 1886, pp. 536–40). A French physician argued for subcutaneous injections of pure carbolic acid, which he argued was largely excreted by the lungs (*Medical Record,* vol. 29, January 30, 1886, p. 128). Another French physician advocated rectal injections of sulphurous gas (*Medical Record,* vol. 30, October 30, 1886, p. 494). Reporting on this, Shrady commented, "Dr. Bergeon's method is novel, and with so many strong endorsements it plainly deserves an extended trial" (*Medical Record,* vol. 31, January 15, 1887, p. 72).

All of this effort to kill the bacillus created controversy. Two schools of physicians were described by Shrady in an editorial: "The one [school] is laboring to find some means of checking phthisis by destroying its supposed parasitic cause; the other still maintains that a constitutional dyscrasia [depraved state] is the main thing for the therapeutists to consider and that attempts to treat this disease by directly destroying the bacilli are futile and impracticable." Shrady believed that most physicians were of the latter view. Quoting Buchner, he wrote:

An infectious disease (and phthisis in most of its forms is surely that) . . . is a battle between body-cells and the micrococci. The result is inflammation and fever. The therapeutist may help the organism in the contest by strengthening the force of the cells, but he cannot destroy or weaken the micrococci without equally injuring the tissues within which they are imbedded. Hence, in phthisis, he recommends nutritive stimulants, not antiseptics. Among the best of these stimulants . . . is arsenic, and this drug seems likely to be brought forward again into prominence in the treatment of phthisis (*Medical Record,* vol. 25, March 1, 1884, p. 238).

Regarding "anti-parasitic treatment" Shrady listed several solutions that did not destroy the bacillus: "sublimate solutions (1:1,000), salicylic acid solutions (1:500), carbolic (1:20), resorcin, solutions of bromine (1:1,000) and oxygenated water" (p. 238). However, he noted that a temperature of 100 to 120 degrees centigrade was sufficient to destroy the bacillus.

Among the inhalants he listed iodoform as most common but cautioned that inhalants "only go a short distance into the bronchi, and never reach the alveoli at all." Shrady concluded, "The antiseptic treatment of phthisis has yet to gain a foothold in therapeutics. While inhalations may occasionally do some good in relieving symptoms and lessening the complicating bronchitis, we must still use our strongest efforts to help the cell rather than kill the bacillus" (pp. 238–39).

Over this period the controversy persisted, and Trudeau's case records reveal many attempts to replicate some of these antiseptic treatments. As he could grow the bacillus and produce tuberculosis by inoculating healthy guinea pigs and rabbits, a logical approach would be to see if he could kill the bacillus, much as Lister had used carbolic acid to kill bacteria on surgical wounds. In a series of experiments lasting several years Trudeau and physician colleagues, who came to cure their tuberculosis but were talked into doing laboratory studies, tried killing the bacilli with every kind of agent imaginable. Not only did they try various agents, but Trudeau's laboratory tested all agents that others felt were effective. Reflecting on these years in a paper delivered at Johns Hopkins, Trudeau wrote:

A good deal of the work of the laboratory has been given to testing experimentally all proposed specific methods of treatment and all consumption cures. The outlook at first seemed to tend toward the application of germicidal substance and many experiments, which all proved barren of results, were made in this direction. We soon learned that the tubercle bacillus bore "cheerfully" a degree of medication which proved fatal to his host. We found that creosote, iodoform, sulphurated hydrogen, hydrofluoric acid, essence of peppermint and other germicides proposed as cures, while they had no influence on the tuberculous process, often tended to shorten the lives of treated animals. The publication of these researches, however, had some influence in disproving the claims of these specifics, and in preventing to a certain extent their more general application to the treatment of the human subject (Trudeau, 1901a).

Trudeau was careful to do these experiments on guinea pigs and rabbits. Two papers reported some of the results. In 1887 he published "Sulphretted Hydrogen versus the Tubercle Bacillus," answering Shrady. For twenty minutes he bathed a pure culture of tubercle bacilli in a closed test tube with undiluted hydrogen sulfide gas. Mixing the contents of the tube with sterilized water he injected the pleural cavities of two rabbits. Although they were well fed and kept in a favorable environment, they both died after 162 days. Their autopsies revealed "typical and advanced pulmonary tuberculosis." Trudeau concluded

This simple experiment seems worthy of record, inasmuch as the evidence it presents may help to correct any false impression already existing as to the germicidal value of H_2S. It also serves to demonstrate the resisting power of the tubercle bacillus and its spores as well as the difficulties attending any attempt at its destruction in living tissues by chemical agents. If so thorough an exposure to the undiluted gas is incapable of destroying this microbe, or of materially staying its destructive power, how futile must be the attempts made to incommode it by rectal injections, or inhalations containing infinitesimal quantities of the apparently feeble agent (Trudeau, 1887b, p. 570).

Trudeau had probably read the writings of Pasteur, who confirmed Koch's work on anthrax. Pasteur had demonstrated that anthrax spores survived in fields where diseased animals had been buried, thus reinfecting more animals. It is likely that he assumed the tubercle bacillus was similarly resistant. The controversy over this treatment continued with additional positive and negative papers, but Trudeau did not continue publishing. As far as he was concerned the controversy had been resolved.

Having attempted hydrofluoric inhalations on at least two of the thirty-five patients treated in 1887 (case # 63 admitted June 16 and case # 71 admitted July 29), Trudeau published "Hydrofluoric Acid as a Destructive Agent to the Tubercle Bacillus" (1888). In a review of the earlier literature he pointed out that "the treatment of phthisis by this chemical compound was suggested to Bastien by the fact that at the glass factories of Baccarat and St. Louis, the vapors of hydrofluoric acid, constantly used in etching, far from injuring the phthisical workmen exposed to them, seemed beneficial to their malady" (p. 486). This treatment was primarily of French origin and may have appealed to him for that reason. He described the chemistry of hydrofluoric acid, noting that the liquid at room temperatures was quite volatile giving off large quantities of whitish fumes, which were highly corrosive and caustic. To make the fumes safe for inhalation Trudeau used what is often referred to in the case records as the "cabinet": "Having made a small room, in which the patient sits, as air-tight as possible, a lead crucible containing one to two teaspoonfuls of the acid is placed in a tin vessel holding hot water, under which an alcohol lamp is kept burning; the amount of vapor evolved will depend on the amount of heat applied, which can be regulated according to the patient's tolerance. The inhalations, when properly diluted, have produced no bad effects in any case, and are not contraindicated even when a tendency to haemoptysis exists" (p. 487).

Dr. Henry Thomas described his experience while a patient: "I saw that he would like to try it on a patient as well as on inoculated animals, and I suggested that I try it on myself. He was somewhat loth to let me do so, but finally consented, and thereafter I sat for two hours a day in a room breathing the fumes of hydrofluoric acid, and with the result that every bit of glass in the room was etched and that the bacilli disappeared from my expectoration. The rabbits did not fare so well, and although one or two other patients tried it, no further results were obtained" (Thomas, 1916, p. 103).

Trudeau described experiments to determine "what destructive power, if any, hydrofluoric acid possesses over the tubercle bacillus." In the first experiment he put virulent tubercle bacilli cultures into 5 cc of hydrofluoric acid in concentrations of 1:100, 1:200, 1:400, 1:800, and 1:1600 and inoculated two rabbits in the right lung to keep as controls. After one hour some bits of bacilli are removed with a platinum needle and planted on two blood-serum tubes, which are labeled and incubated. The remaining bacilli settle, and the acid is drawn off. Sterilized water is mixed with the bacilli, and 2 cc of each solution is injected into the right lung of two healthy rabbits. The two rabbits used as controls died as expected, proving that the bacilli were virulent. Two animals injected from the 1:100 and 1:200 solutions died, also. However, as no bacilli could be found, Trudeau assumed it was because they were injected with the full acid solution, before the acid was drawn off. The "deaths were due solely to the corrosive action of the acid." The remaining animals did not die, and Trudeau concluded that solutions of hydrofluoric acid between 1:400 and 1:800 effectively killed the virulent tubercle bacilli.

To illustrate the clarity of Trudeau's descriptions the second experiment will be presented as it appeared.

Acidulated Air

Experiment II.—December 18, 1887. A small bit of linen cloth attached to a platinum wire is first sterilized, then dipped on the condensation water of a tube containing a culture of the tubercle bacillus, and rubbed over the germs growing on the surface of the serum. It is then withdrawn, and from it two tubes planted in the usual way, and kept as controls. The wire with its rag is then inserted into a small round cylinder, corked at both ends with cotton wadding. Through this cylinder a current of atmospheric air, previously allowed to bubble through a 1:3 solution of hydrofluoric acid and water, held in a gutta-percha bottle is steadily passed for one hour, the necessary pressure being obtained from a compressed air apparatus attached to the gutta-percha bottle. At the end of an hour the wire and rag are withdrawn and rubbed on the surface of four solidified serum tubes. These, together with the controls, are put in the thermostat.

January 18. The controls are covered with growth, while the other tubes have remained sterile.

January 20. The surface of the sterile tubes is scraped, and replants made from all of them.

February 14. No growth has appeared in any of the replants.

This experiment was repeated a month later, with the same results (Trudeau, 1888, pp. 487–88).

These results showed that acidulated air (air containing hydrofluoric acid) killed the tubercle bacillus.

In the third experiment Trudeau bubbled the same acidulated air through tubes containing virulent bacilli mixed in sterilized water. After an hour the bacilli were used to plant cultures and inject the right lung of three rabbits. The control rabbits showed tuberculosis, while all three experimental rabbits were normal. This provided more evidence that acidulated air could kill the bacillus.

In the fourth experiment he subjected serum tubes containing cultures of the tubercle bacillus to "a current of air previously passed through a 1:5 solution of hydrofluoric acid in water . . . directed through a glass pipette into each tube for half an hour." The tubes showed no growth of tubercle bacilli, while controls showed growth. The experiment was repeated using dilutions of 1:7, 1:9, 1:16, 1:30, and 1:50. At a concentration of 1:50 the acidulated air did not appear to kill the bacilli.

In the next experiment, Trudeau dipped a "rag attached to a platinum wire" into blood containing the bacillus. Two control tubes were planted using the rag, which was then placed under a 1,500 cc bell-jar. Also under the jar he placed "0.20 of hydrofluoric acid" on a sheet of lead. With gentle heat the acid was vaporized for one hour. The rag was then used to plant three liquid serum tubes. The two controls showed growth of bacilli, while the three experimental serum tubes had no growth. He repeated this using 0.15 of hydrofluoric acid, but this time the experimental tubes showed growth of bacilli also. Trudeau concluded: "one part of acid, vaporized in 7,500 of air, is the smallest quantity that will effectually destroy putrefactive bacteria after an hour's exposure."

Finally Trudeau inoculated virulent bacilli into four rabbits in the right lung and the "anterior chamber of the right eye." Two were placed in an airtight box for three hours every day into which acidulated air was introduced. All four rabbits developed tuberculosis in the inoculated eye. Both of the controls were killed and showed "the usual appearances of advanced pulmonary tuberculosis." Compared to the controls, the two rabbits that had inhaled acidulated air showed local tubercle at the point of inoculation but less elsewhere in the lungs. Trudeau concluded, "In comparing the autopsies all that can be said is that whereas no difference exists in the extent and character of the pleural disease, less tubercle has invaded the lung tissue proper in the animals subjected to the inhalations. The direction taken by the disease might in so small a number of cases be purely accidental, and no satisfactory conclusion can be arrived at from the result of this experiment, the proof being insufficient and of a somewhat uncertain character" (Trudeau, 1888, p. 489).

From the five experiments Trudeau concluded that hydrofluoric acid could destroy the tubercle bacillus:

In the treatment of the existing lesions of pulmonary phthisis the hydrofluoric inhalations would at least possess over the antiseptic sprays, already in use, the advantages of tested efficiency and greater penetrability. It is evident, however, that even if the acidulated air could be breathed without injurious effects in dilutions which have been found to be efficient, but a small proportion of the bacilli, namely, those lying directly in contact with the atmospheric air, could thereby be destroyed while no antagonistic effect on those imbedded in solidified areas of lung, tubercular nodules, or diseased glands could be hoped for.

An excellent illustration of the inefficiency of antiseptics beyond their point of actual contact is given by the autopsies in Experiment VI, which showed the course of the tubercular pleurisy to have been entirely uninfluenced by the daily inhalations to which the animals were subjected. . . .

It is not likely that hydrofluoric acid can alter those chemical and vital changes in the organism which allow of the growth of this microbe, and to this end thus far those conditions which promote bodily vigor have alone been found effectual. The recommendations of the method, however, are that its application is easy and does not interfere with the employment of hygienic and climatic treatment, and that by it we may hope to diminish the amount of virus against which the organism has to contend. Whether this hope will be realized, an extended clinical application of the treatment alone can determine (Trudeau, 1888, pp. 489–90).

After publishing this article Trudeau used hydrofluoric acid inhalations quite sparingly. Patient # 107, labeled a "hopeless case," admitted July 4, 1888, took "hydrofluoric acid every day," but the record does not indicate whether this was by inhalation in the Cabinet. After this patient Trudeau continued inhalation in the Cabinet but switched to creosote (case # 131, admitted October 21; case # 134, admitted October 22; case # 139, admitted December 18; and case # 141, admitted December 27).

The clearly described and carefully analyzed animal experiments were done in the small laboratory room attached to Trudeau's home. He did much of the research during the winter, probably as an interesting way to spend the long cold months. Each spring he would emerge with some results to be presented at the meetings of the American Climatological Association or the Association of American Physicians. These would automatically get published in the *Transactions of the American Climatological Association* or get picked up by one of the physicians editing a medical journal. Dr. George Gould published the *Medical News* and was a good friend of Trudeau. Dr. George Shrady published the *Medical Record* and his friendship with Trudeau was strained because he was slow to support mandatory isolation of tuberculosis patients. Publicity from these publications established Trudeau's credentials as a careful, cautious researcher who based his conclusions on the results derived from experiment. These scientific methods brought a refreshing new approach to a profession that had relied for so long on the personal testimonies of doctors whose objectivity may have been quite limited by their self-interest. As a result Trudeau came to be respected as someone who would evaluate a treatment carefully and present the results fairly.

Because he was isolated in the mountains, Trudeau did not have affiliations that could have put his objectivity in question. Therefore he was sent a variety of things to test. For example, George M. Sternberg, now of the Surgeon General's Office, War Department, Washington, sent Trudeau a translation of a letter he received from Dr. Carasso, Director of the Military Hospital in Genoa, Italy. Since 1888 Carasso had experimented with

continuous inhalation of the essential oil of peppermint and, at the same time, in the administration by the mouth of an alcoholic solution of creosote with glycerine and chloroform, to which is added the essential oil of peppermint in the proportion of one percent. This treatment has been attended with the most brilliant results, inasmuch as we have obtained cure not only of all cases of Pulmonary tuberculosis in the first state but also in the more advanced stages with ample and numerous cavities and with the presence of numerous bacilli in the sputa.

Sternberg commented: "If you think this matter worthy of investigation I shall be glad to know the results of your clinical experiments" (December 30, 1893, correspondence). Evidently this was investigated by E. R. Baldwin, who published an unenthusiastic article, "The Effect of Peppermint Inhalation on Experimental Tuberculosis," in the *New York Medical Journal*, vol. 61, 1895, p. 623.

Using electricity, inventors created technologies and sent advertisements of devices that the laboratory did not test. In 1894, J. C. Dittrich of New York City sent a drawing of his "ozone machine, which is capable of producing ozone in sufficient quantity for therapeutic purposes." He legitimated his claim by mentioning the names of several doctors who used it "with the most satisfactory results" and mentioned a large ozone machine requiring electric current, which was "used to ozonize the atmosphere in a large room of patients" (February 8, 1894, correspondence). Robert Casey, A.B., of Denver wrote Trudeau, describing "The Robert Casey Electro-Inhalent Consumption Cure":

a powerful, penetrating antiseptic gas is generated from chemicals treated by discharge through them of a flash of Static Electricity . . . a Subtle, Depurating [cleansing], Balsamic Gas . . . Deeply and slowly inspired, that gas attacks and begins to decompose the pus, slimes and tubercular matter filling the small bronchi and cells of the lungs. It quickly changes them into a fermenting watery state, easy to expectorate. And in doing this, it completely sterilizes the matter so attacked. The action is strictly chemical, and is indispensable to any real cure for the disease (Casey, 1895, correspondence, p. 14).

Given what Trudeau had written about ozone in the woods, this enterprising inventor probably thought he could get medical support from the doctor. Evidently these devices were not tested in the laboratory perhaps because they were recommended by engineers, not doctors, or more likely because electricity was not available until 1895 at Saranac Lake.

To use an antiseptic to kill the bacillus remained a goal for Trudeau. After all, the acidulated hydrofluoric acid did kill the bacteria in the test tube. Inhalation was still a popular form of treatment, and after Trudeau's papers others were published continuing to advocate iodoform inhalations and sulfuretted hydrogen (*Journal of Medical Sciences,* vol. 95, January 1888, pp. 394–95) and inhalation of sulphurous acid gas (*American Journal of Medical Sciences,* vol. 95, January 1888, p. 508).

Shrady commented on this latter article, "The French are so intensely enthusiastic over everything that seems to promise good results, that they are apt to rush into print before their theories are fully justified by facts. This treatment can, of course, only be carried on in hospitals, and it is to be hoped that equally good reports may be heard later, and that it may not share the fate of the rectal injection method" (*Medical Record,* vol. 33, March 31, 1888, p. 358).

Others argued for inhalation of pure oxygen and ozonized oxygen (*American Journal of Medical Sciences,* vol. 96, August 1888, pp. 182–83); hydrofluoric acid (*Journal of Medical Sciences,* vol. 96, October 1888, p. 409); inhalations of aniline oil (*Medical Record,* vol. 33, June 2, 1888, p. 610); inhalations of hot air (*Medical Record,* vol. 34, October 27, 1888, pp. 511–12); inhalations in general (*Medical Record,* vol. 34, November 24, 1888, p. 621); hot moist inhalations (*Medical Record,* vol. 34, December 1, 1888, p. 660); formulae for drugs by atomization (*Medical News,* vol. 52, March 17, 1888, p. 295); cold air inhalations (*Medical News,* vol. 53, August 4, 1888, p. 130); and hot air inhalations (*Medical News,* vol. 53, October 20, 1888, p. 446). Often these papers just noted that patients improved, but without controls there was no evidence that the inhalation had made a difference. Others said there was a decrease of bacilli in the sputum, but without an adequate way to measure the amount of bacilli in the sputum, this result was suspect, also. Although these articles claimed to be scientific, they were essentially extensions of the old empirical method of clinical medicine. "I tried this and got good results, therefore, I testify to its value." Experiments using control groups were where science was going, but most clinicians had not grasped that idea.

One paper confirmed Trudeau's findings on hydrofluoric acid. After injecting animals with the bacillus and treating some by inhalation, it was observed that those treated by inhalation lived longer but were still tubercular. The authors concluded that "The idea of killing the bacilli within the human body by the inhalation of hydrofluoric acid cannot be entertained, but the possibility of weakening or even destroying their virulence, must be admitted" (*American Journal of the Medical Sciences,* vol. 96, December 1888, p. 623). Shrady concluded that experimental evidence showed it was doubtful that inhalations of these vapors are curative, but they might weaken the bacilli and therefore aid "the tissues in their struggle against the ravages of the invader" (*Medical Record,* vol. 34, September 1, 1888, pp. 247–48).

On December 15, 1888, the *Medical Record* carried a paper by Dr. Louis Weigert of Berlin, who had developed an apparatus that heated air, allowing patients to inhale hot air through a mouthpiece. On the basis of five cases he claimed "in most cases, a complete cessation of the acute process within a short time" (Weigert, 1888, pp. 693–95). Evidently Weigert marketed his apparatus and made advertising claims that were not appreciated. One of Trudeau's friends, Dr. A. Jacobi, read a paper before the New York Academy of Medicine in which he asserted that, contrary to advertising claims made by Weigert, he had not "bought, endorsed or recommended" the apparatus for hot air inhalations in treatment of tuberculosis. Jacobi had used the apparatus along with other physicians at Bellevue Hospital, but after an initial favorable impression he was now of the opinion that it was not useful and might be injurious to some patients (*Medical Record,* vol. 36, no. 2, July 13, 1889, p. 53). Before the American Medical Association a Dr. E. L. Shirley of Detroit reported on eight cases in which he used the Weigert apparatus. In five of the cases treatment had to be discontinued because of discomfort or negative effects. Three cases had positive results (*Medical Record,* vol. 36, no. 1, July 8, 1889, p. 25).

Having read these inconclusive articles about the inhalation of hot air and perhaps wanting to support his fellow members, Trudeau read a paper before the Association of American Physicians on September 20, 1889, describing four cases (Trudeau, 1889, pp. 337–38). The question he was investigating was: "Are inhalations of dry hot air capable of preventing the growth of the bacillus tuberculosis in the lungs of living individuals, or of diminishing the virulence of this microbe?" (p. 337). The patients were quickly increased to four hours of inhalation daily, divided into two sessions. Temperature of the air measured by a thermometer on the mouthpiece was 200 degrees centigrade (392 degrees fahrenheit). Two patients showed slight improvements in their symptoms but could not be convinced to continue. A third patient continued for "over three months" but with no improvement. The fourth patient (case # 144, January 8, 1889) improved after three months but then lost ground. Trudeau concluded, "This brief clinical study does not furnish evidence which differs materially from that usually obtained on the trial of many specific methods of treatment for tuberculosis hitherto put forward and long ago abandoned. The improvement which manifested itself in one case, though marked, was no greater than was observed to occur at the same time, from climatic and hygienic treatment alone, in several of the men's fellow patients" (p. 338). In all four cases the sputum was examined before treatment and every five weeks during treatment. "In every instance bacilli were found." Inhalation did not eliminate the bacilli.

Next, he devised a way to test whether the virulence of the bacilli decreased as a result of inhaling hot air.

Before beginning the inhalations a small portion of the sputum from Case IV was mixed with sterilized water and injected into the thoracic cavity of three rabbits. The animals were killed five weeks later and a localized tubercular lesion at the site of injection was noted, while transparent miliary tubercles were just visible on the pleura and pericardium. These lesions contained bacilli. The patient having begun to breathe hot air for four hours daily, a small portion of his expectoration was taken every five weeks and injected in the same manner into the thoracic cavity of three rabbits. This was repeated three times—that is, the last set of inoculations was made three months and a half after the treatment had begun. Each set of rabbits was killed at intervals of five weeks and notes of the autopsies made. They were found to have all developed tubercular lesions containing bacilli, and in the last lot as well as in the others, miliary tubercles occuring at some distance from the site of injection were demonstrated. These tubercles were sufficiently advanced to be macroscopical, and did not differ materially in their appearance from those which had been produced in the animals inoculated with material expectorated by this man before the treatment was instituted. Five weeks being very nearly the earliest date at which secondary tubercle distant from the original lesion appears, microbes capable of causing such manifestations within this limited time can have lost none of their virulence. No diminution in the pathogenic properties of the bacilli seems therefore to have been produced by breathing the heated air (p. 338).

Observing no decrease in the ability of the bacilli to produce the disease in rabbits' lungs, Trudeau was satisfied that hot-air inhalation did not decrease virulence. Then he attempted to explain this finding from his knowledge of lung anatomy.

Although difficult of absolute demonstration, it is most probable that the temperature of the air-cell itself can be influenced but very slightly, no matter how high or how low that of the inspired air may prove to be. The intense vascularity of the lungs, the fixed temperature of the blood rapidly circulating through them (which is relatively low when compared to that of the heated atmosphere furnished by the apparatus), the moisture and infinite subdivision of the surfaces, and the very slow admixture which takes place between the tidal and residual air, all conspire to rob the incoming current of its heat and to confine the possible variations of temperature in the air-cell within very narrow limits.

The inference held out as conclusive that, because the breath on expiration measures as high as 45 degree centigrade (113 degrees fahrenheit), the air in the air cells must necessarily be much warmer is fallacious, for the expired air is in a great part composed of the last inspiration still surcharged with its recently acquired heat. As the bacilli in the bronchial secretions must necessarily be brought in much more intimate contact with the hot air than those imbedded in solidified areas of lung or in impermeable tubercular masses, the failure of the latter agent to diminish their virulence to any appreciable degree is most significant (p. 338).

Because it was read before the Association of American Physicians this paper had considerable prestige. It was published eight days later in *Medical News,* September 28, 1889, and reported by Shrady in the *Medical Record* of the same date (p. 356).

CREOSOTE TREATMENTS

The next trend that developed was the use of creosote to destroy the bacillus. Dr. Beverley Robinson (1889) argued that patients improved most rapidly with the joint treatment of antiseptic inhalations of creosote and creosote in gelatin capsules given internally with cod liver oil after meals. In the *Medical Record* Shrady noted that both Beverley Robinson and Austin Flint had reported alleviation of symptoms particularly in incipient cases but neither reported on the presence of bacilli. He concluded, "from what has been written on the creosote treatment of phthisis, we may feel reasonably certain that the remedy is not devoid of utility in its proper sphere. The climatic treatment of consumption is, after all, but the rich man's remedy. By far the larger number of phthisical patients will continue to seek relief from their ailments by the use of medicines, and creosote will doubtless soon be employed on a sufficiently large scale to definitely determine its true value" (*Medical Record,* vol. 35, no. 2, January 12, 1859, p. 45).

This would have been a natural topic for Trudeau to study. He began to use creosote in 1887 in the Cabinet for inhalations and in pill form as well (case # 58, admitted May 23, 1887). It was used in 1888, and more frequently in 1889. For example in 1889 of seventy-two patients treated, fifty-three or 74 percent received creosote in some form. The case records are not clear about the form in which creosote was used. Usually the record reads "Rx: creosote." When it read "creosote and brandy," "creosote and cod liver oil," or "creosote and antifebrin," we can assume it was given internally. How often the Cabinet was used for inhaling is unclear.

More articles praising creosote appeared (*Medical Record,* vol. 35, no. 8, May 4, 1889, pp. 483–84; vol. 36, no. 6, August 10, 1889, p. 145; vol. 37, no. 13, March 29, 1890, p. 353). In the fall of 1890 came the first warning that administration of creosote might be associated with renal irritation and perhaps kidney disease (*American Journal of the Medical Sciences,* vol. 100, no. 5, November 1890, p. 501). Soon after these warnings Trudeau decreased its use. In 1890 the frequency of use decelerated, and by the summer of 1891 creosote does not appear in the case records. Trudeau seemed to follow trends as long as people he trusted recommended them, but at the first indication of harm to patients he easily got off the bandwagon. By 1890 he would have had enough clinical experience with the drug to make his own judgment.

PREVENTION—ISOLATION

Another phase of laboratory work supported the public health movement, which had gained respect by preventing a cholera outbreak in New York City after the Civil War (Rosenberg, 1962, p. 213f). Once Koch's findings were accepted in this country, public health officials did what they could to prevent the spread of tuberculosis. A resident physician at the sanitarium did studies of the dust in tenements, rooms of consumptives, and railroad cars. When guinea pigs were inoculated with this dust they died of tuberculosis, suggesting that the dust carried the bacilli. His paper concluded: "It shows that the seed sown by the board of health in its efforts to enforce compulsory notification of tuberculosis cases and subsequent disinfection and renovation of quarters occupied by such people is bearing good fruit, since all four of the cleanly apartments were free from infection." The paper argued for the cleaning of elevated railroad cars, removal of dried sputum, preventing people from spitting on the street, and the development of state hospitals for tuberculosis patients (Hance, 1897).

Another argument still persisted in the literature. It is interesting because it parallels arguments being made today about how to treat AIDS patients. In 1889 the move began to classify tuberculosis as a contagious disease and to legalize public health methods of prevention. Up to this time deaths from eight contagious diseases were routinely reported by doctors. These included typhus fever, typhoid fever, scarlet fever, cerebrospinal meningitis, measles, diphtheria, smallpox, and yellow fever. Each month the *Medical Record* contained a tally of new cases reported to the New York City Health Department. As some of the clinical physicians had caught up with the bacteriologists, tuberculosis could now be certified as a contagious disease, reported by physicians, and appropriate preventive policies and procedures instituted. Before the Connecticut State Medical Society, Dr. Seth Hills, said, "It was time . . . for the medical profession to take some decisive action in regard to tuberculosis. Why was the typhoid-fever germ hunted to its death and the germ of consumption, that most widespread of germ diseases, allowed to go scot-free?" (*Medical Record,* vol. 35, no. 23, June 8, 1889, p. 641). He advocated isolation of consumptives from the healthy. In an editorial, Dr. Shrady argued for classifying tuberculosis with the contagious diseases reported to the New York City Health Department. "The advantages of this step would be that it would educate both physician and public to the view that phthisis is infectious. . . . On the other hand, it might needlessly alarm the public and perhaps add, unnecessarily, to the discomfort and suffering of the patients" (*Medical Record,* vol. 36, no. 2, July 13, 1889, p. 44).

Shrady and others expressed concern about the wholesale isolation of all consumptives. First of all, this would be a logistical nightmare, as there were not enough facilities to accommodate everyone. This may have been part of the reason physicians were reluctant to label tuberculosis contagious. Second, physicians were concerned about the social effect of stigmatizing by labeling large numbers of patients who are not very contagious. Underlying these two concerns was the fear that they might lose their patients to other facilities. Third, the contagion was somewhat unique. Because it was transmitted by the sputum of consumptives finding its way to particularly susceptible people, control of expectoration became the problem. This method of transmission called for a campaign of prevention.

The New York City Board of Health issued a list of rules, in July 1889, to prevent the spread of consumption. The rules were written by Hermann Biggs in consultation with T. M. Prudden and H. P. Loomis (Lowell, 1969, p. 10). They stated that because in the usual way of transmission the germs are suspended as dust in the air breathed from the dried sputa of consumptives, their policy intended to minimize this possibility. Consumptives were not allowed to spit on the floor or into a cloth, but they were to spit into a bowl with 1:1000 corrosive sublimate [mercuric chloride, an antiseptic]. Their rooms were to have minimal furnishings, bare floors, and the like. The Board of Health also passed a resolution requiring the reporting of deaths from tuberculosis (*Medical Record,* vol. 36, no. 2, July 13, 1889, p. 45). Similar ideas were discussed at the seventeenth annual meeting of the Public Health Association (*Medical Record,* vol. 36, no. 18, November 2, 1889, p. 499). These general policies were accepted, though physicians differed over specifics, such as whether corrosive sublimate could destroy the bacillus (*Medical Record,* vol. 36, no. 3, July 20, 1889, p. 79), how to disinfect rooms (*Medical Record,* vol. 36, no. 17, October 26, 1889, p. 464), and the best design for a "sputum flask." Trudeau had suggested a flask made of cardboard that could be burned. It was preferred over a spittoon that must be washed (*Medical Record,* vol. 37, no. 6, February 8, 1890, p. 159). The New York City Health Department issued "Information for Consumptives and Those Living with Them" on February 13, 1894, in English, German, Hebrew, and Italian. The pamphlet warned that tuberculosis was contagious and sputum the chief agent. It suggested that all sputum be burned and rooms of consumptives carefully cleaned. The names of people suffering with consumption were to be reported to the Health Department so that a doctor could be sent to examine them.

As the isolation of consumptives became accepted, physicians were very concerned about the impact upon individuals. They did not want these people to be stigmatized to such an extent that they would be rejected like lepers by society or their families. Reporting on a meeting at the Paris Academy of Medicine, Shrady's correspondent wrote, "There was also concern about emphasizing contagiousness and needlessly frightening the public and causing unnecessary avoidance of phthisical patients. They emphasized that practice of good hygiene by all was the most important factor" (*Medical Record,* vol. 36, no. 11, September 14, 1889, p. 306). It was about this time that the scientific community began to use the word "tuberculosis" to refer to the disease caused by the tubercle bacillus. The old words, "consumption" and "phthisis," slowly disappeared from the medical vocabulary. Whether changing the name lessened the stigma attached to the diagnostic label is not known (*American Journal of Medical Sciences,* vol. 49, January 1890, pp. 78–79).

Shrady advocated special hospitals for consumptives not just to isolate them but because "the treatment of phthisis, if properly carried out, requires much attention and skill, and the employment often of special apparatus" (*Medical Record,* vol. 36, no. 24, December 7, 1889, p. 634). He recommended that city hospitals have country branches where they could send curable cases. The idea of special hospitals was argued at the fifth annual meeting of the Association of American Physicians in Philadelphia by E. O. Shakespeare. E. L. Trudeau supported the suggestion (*Medical Record,* vol. 37, no. 21, May 24, 1890, p. 598).

Early in 1890 Trudeau published a brief letter in *Medical News* supporting the idea of quarantine in general. When a case of influenza was discovered in the village of Sarance Lake, Trudeau immediately quarantined the Adirondack Cottage Sanitarium because he feared "an attack of the prevalent influenza might prove disastrous to many of the 'invalids' residing there." While the epidemic attacked the majority of the people in the surrounding community no cases appeared at the sanitarium (*Medical News,* February 15, 1890, pp. 185–86).

STATISTICS AND PREJUDICE

Another result of this emphasis upon prevention was the use of statistics to focus preventive efforts on specific communities with high mortality. Dr. F. B. Westbrook gave a paper at the New York Academy of Medicine stating that the greater mortality from phthisis in cities was the result of preventable conditions like defective sewage systems, crowded work conditions, and low-grade tenement housing. Also, he made the biased argument that the many immigrants in the city were more susceptible by nature. After citing mortality rates varying from 1.203 to 9.71 per thousand, Westbrook said, "The causes of these wide variations were the character of the location as regards soil and drainage, the presence or absence of the worst class of tenements. The presence of public institutions, particularly hospitals, and the nationality of the inhabitants" (*Medical Record,* vol. 37, no. 2, March 22, 1890, p. 334). The discussant for this paper was Dr. A. L. Loomis, who urged caution in interpreting these statistics but agreed, saying that they "proved simply that under unhygienic conditions the death-rate from phthisis was higher than under good hygienic conditions. They went a little further, also, and showed that the descendants of certain races offered greater power of resistance to tubercular disease than those of others" (p. 335). Loomis suggested that the city provided more chance of infection, especially in tenement-house areas.

Shrady contributed to these prejudiced ideas in an editorial commenting on a paper comparing consumption mortality rates of people of American-born parentage versus individuals who were foreign-born. Dr. Hurd argued that lower rates among American born showed that they had developed an acquired immunity. Shrady, however, pointed to the sociological factors, noting that immigrants were less well fed and housed, living under poorer hygienic conditions. Nevertheless he went on, ignoring these facts, to perpetuate his prejudice. "If the mortality rate from phthisis is increasing among them, it is largely because of the well known fact that we are getting a much lower grade of immigrant than we used to receive" (*Medical Record,* vol. 36, no. 6, August 10, 1889, p. 154). This emphasis upon nationality differences in the face of glaring socioeconomic differences illustrates the depth of ethnic prejudice. Hand washing, frequent bathing, and the use of soap were new hygienic practices that were just becoming popular and were largely confined to the upper social classes, who could afford soap and running water. But the massive flood of immigrants attracted to cities by industrial expansion could not afford these luxuries.

By 1890 tuberculosis was widely accepted as a contagious disease. When physicians accepted the idea of contagion, they were forced to look at the sources and contexts of contagion, which were primarily the deplorable living and working conditions of poor people. Though public health measures could be used to change these inhuman conditions, there were economic and political powers who resisted spending funds to help these immigrant populations. Therefore, the focus of prevention was not primarily on changing the social conditions that encouraged poor hygiene and increased people's susceptiblity to the disease. Though efforts and some progress were made in this direction, prevention focused on individuals, urging people to adopt hygienic habits and isolating the carriers of the disease. But without soap and water available these individual efforts are useless. This dilemma is constantly faced by public health workers. Unfortunately political and economic powers nearly always preclude attacking the health problem at the social level (housing, clean water, and sewers), where the effect would be greater and more permanent.

9

Search for a Vaccine

Building on his earlier attempts to destroy the bacillus Trudeau gave another paper to the Association of American Physicians on some basic research that he hoped would provide knowledge leading to a vaccine similar to that already developed for anthrax. He compared two cultures that appeared somewhat different. The first culture had been obtained from his friend Prudden, at the College of Physicians and Surgeons, who had taken it "from the lung of a man dead of acute miliary Tuberculosis." Trudeau grew it for three generations and noted that "it grew very slowly in very dry, isolated, and heaped scaly masses." The second culture

was obtained from the lesions of a guinea-pig dead from general tuberculosis induced by inoculation of a small amount of material taken from an old phthisical cavity. This culture was brought from France by Dr. G. Currier, and has been under cultivation for a long time, being occasionally allowed almost to die out before being replanted. Its gross appearance is entirely different from No. 1. It grows more rapidly in an even film which, toward the end of the third week, begins, to raise in high irregular pleats above the level of the culture medium. It is nowhere dry or scaly, but is moist and of consistency of very thick cream (Trudeau, 1890b, pp. 183–84).

Comparing the cultures under the microscope he noted: "these two cultures differ only in that the rods in No. 2 are a trifle shorter and broader than in No. 1" (p. 104). Then he compared the virulence of the two cultures. Observing that they were different he inoculated groups of rabbits and noted that No. 1 was "more rapidly fatal to life." No. 2 killed only "one animal out of fifteen within three months" (p. 184). After making plants in glycerine agar from the tubercles in the rabbits, he noted that the microscopic differences in the two cultures persisted. Trudeau concluded:

As far as I am aware, this is the first record of any variation capable of being reproduced which has been noted in the tubercle bacillus. In other bacteria, in anthrax notably, wide variations of growth and virulence can be brought about at will; and the interest which attaches to the facts I present is that it is through these variations that vaccine for anthrax and other microbic diseases has been discovered, enabling the experimenter to produce for those diseases a microbe possessing the protective power of the virulent germ without its deadly pathogenic properties (p. 184).

Much of this paper (1890b) was repeated in an invited presentation Trudeau gave before the New York Pathological Society (1891). After displaying the different cultures he had obtained from Dr. Prudden and Dr. Currier and repeating the information in the earlier paper, he exhibited and described "several flasks containing a pure culture of the tubercle bacillus in a liquid medium." Finally he showed "two sets of lungs taken from rabbits inoculated in the rim of the ear with a pure culture of tubercle bacillus, and killed two and three and a half months respectively after the inoculation" (p. 17). He pointed out that both sets of lungs "presented the same lesions, but at different stages. . . . They were both literally riddled with tubercular nodules, and large caseating foci were pretty evenly distributed on the pleural surface. These large caseous masses may have been produced at the spots where small lumps of culture have become lodged" (p. 77). He concluded by showing a third set of lungs taken from a rabbit ten weeks after inoculation with the live bacillus "into the right pleura and lung." This rabbit had been "kept out of doors and under excellent hygienic conditions." These lungs were quite different from the two sets of lungs just displayed.

No microscopical tubercles are seen in this case to stud the lung and pleura, but several large, fibrous-looking tumors, adherent to the visceral pleura, are visible at the point of injection and at various other places on the surface of the lung and pericardium. These gigantic nodules are seen to consist, of a thick fibrous capsule containing a mass of caseous material swarming with bacilli (p. 77).

He showed a drawing of a microscopic picture done by Dr. Prudden, which illustrated "the encapsulated bacilli in the center of a very thick fibrous capsule which ends in a narrow pedicle attached to the plural surface. The bacilli swarm in the center, diminish in numbers as the capsule is approached, and not a single one is to be seen in the fibrous tissue of which the latter is composed" (p. 77).

This information would have been interesting to the members of the pathological society because they were learning and teaching the new science of bacteriology also. The display of Prudden's drawing illustrated Trudeau's theory of what an outdoor life in the woods could do for someone with tuberculosis. He believed that rest, fresh air, and good nutrition encouraged this encapsulating process. "What would have been the subsequent fate of these microbes thus imprisoned can only be a matter of conjecture, but it does not seem unlikely that they would ultimately have been obliterated by the steady contraction of the fibrous tissue surrounding them" (p. 7). Trudeau explained that, in a relapse of tuberculosis, the fibrous capsule broke down, allowing the bacilli to escape and infect the surrounding tissues. He noted that he had obtained "pure cultures of the bacillus, a year after inoculation, from similar nodules taken from the same animal who furnished the specimen for this drawing and who was apparently in good health and presented otherwise sound organs when killed" (pp. 77–78). In the next year he explained this process (Trudeau, 1892a):

We must usually content ourselves with placing our patients amid the most favorable environment attainable, the beneficial influence of which is primarily aimed at the existing malnutrition, and secondarily at the diseased processes; but even if we succeed in arresting the progress of the malady by these means, and in improving nutrition, the patient still carries for a long time an infectious, though dormant element, ready, like a smoldering fire, to break out, and sooner or later, again overcome the newly-acquired resistance (p. 298).

This was related to the research he published in the fall of 1890. The idea of a vaccine that could be used to prevent tuberculosis was foremost in the minds of medical scientists. If tuberculosis was a contagious disease, like cholera, smallpox, anthrax, diphtheria, typhus, and others, then the same methods that Pasteur and Koch had used to develop antitoxins might be productive.

ATTEMPTS TO IMMUNIZE ANIMALS

By this time Trudeau had given up his search for a germicidal for "the direct destruction of the tubercle bacillus in the tissues of man and animals." His attention was focused on the "mysterious powers of resistance" of humans. He felt that "the most promise at present seems to lie in the study of nature's laws of immunity and in learning how far we may influence and imitate these." Trudeau expressed the following opinion:

There appears to be, therefore, over and above the element of physical vigor, a natural immunity against natural means of infection in tuberculosis, as in all other infectious diseases—an immunity possessed to a different degree by different individuals and species of animals, and which is quite sufficient for their protection, no matter at how low an ebb their physical vigor may chance to be whether we believe that immunity is due to the germicidal power of blood serum, or to the phagocytic activity of the cells, to purely chemical reactions intimately connected with the biological life of the tissues, to an insusceptibility of the nerve-centers to the poisonous products of the microbes to a combination of these elements, or to some factor as yet unknown, it is evident that the margin between immunity and susceptibility is a very narrow one at first, that some trifling chemical or biological variation in the tissues is capable of turning the scales for or against infection, and some hope would seem to lie in the possibility of artificially inducing this condition of resistance in them (Trudeau, 1890, p. 565).

Taking encouragement from the work of Pasteur, Trudeau asked, "Can the tubercle bacillus, or the soluble products of its life history, when treated according to the teachings of modern science, be made to confer any degree of immunity against this disease?" (p. 566).

In the first series of experiments, which he labeled "Inoculation of Chemical Substances," three groups of rabbits received inoculations. The first group of five rabbits received *dead surface cultures*: "on three occasions at intervals of four days, subcutaneously, 4 c.c. of *dead* surface culture suspended in distilled water in sufficient amount to make an opaque turbid emulsion" (p. 566). After six or seven weeks, when the rabbits showed no signs of tuberculosis, they were "injected in the lung with ½ c.c. of slightly milky emulsion of *living virulent* tubercle bacilli."

The second group of five rabbits received steam *sterilized liquid* cultures:

These injections are repeated on five occasions, at intervals of five days, increasing gradually the amount to 12 c.c. to each animal. The subcutaneous introduction of this liquid was followed by a marked rise of temperature and by a trifling, but temporary, irritation at the site of puncture; not a single abscess occurred, and the rabbits, when inoculated with virulent culture four weeks from the last vaccination, were apparently in good condition (p. 566).

The third group of five rabbits received *filtered cultures*. The same pure live cultures from the second group were

filtered with very slight pressure through a porcelain Pasteur filter. The clear filtrate proved free from germs, as shown when planted in fresh bouillon tubes, and two animals injected with this liquid and killed three months later presented no tubercular lesions. Injections of this filtered fluid, in the same amounts and at the same intervals as in the preceding lot of animals, were made in five rabbits (p. 566).

These rabbits showed the same elevations in temperature as group two, leading Trudeau to conclude that "the peptones and salts contained in the bouillon" may have caused the temperature increase. But the rabbits in group three were in excellent health without disease and were inoculated with living virulent tubercle bacilli two weeks after their last injection.

A fourth group of five rabbits was inoculated with *living bacilli* and used as controls. After two months the controls were killed, and autopsies of the three groups of rabbits were performed. "All the rabbits are more or less tubercular; the lesions of those in whom this preventive inoculation was practiced differ from those observed in the controls but little" (p. 566). The use of dead surface cultures, sterilized liquid cultures, and filtered cultures did not produce immunity in the rabbits.

Next Trudeau used the bacillus he had described that spring to the Association of American Physicians—culture number 2, which had come from France and appeared less virulent. He had observed that

Rabbits inoculated subcutaneously with these cultures present after four months only an indolent localized lesion at the site of injection and no visceral disease. The cheesy abscess this caused often grows to great size and shows no tendency to open externally; as time goes on it generally loses its cheesy character, becomes gelatinous in appearance and tends often slowly to disappear, the animal still continuing free from visceral disease. Intrapulmonary injections of small amounts produce in rabbits a localized tubercular process with little tendency to spread, or spreading very slowly in rare cases, and which is often entirely recovered from. Intravenous injections of moderate amounts of this attenuated germ gives rise to no appreciable disease, while intra-peritoneal inoculation of large quantities is usually fatal (p. 567).

These results suggested to Trudeau that the bacilli had become attenuated, their virulence "enfeebled." He decided to use cultures of bacilli No. 2 in experiments.

Four guinea pigs were injected subcutaneously in the belly with an "old liquid culture" of these attenuated bacilli. After a week they were injected again with a "fresher culture of a month's growth." Five weeks later the four "appeared in excellent condition," except for "a small unopened abscess at the site of the second preventive inoculation." These four were divided into two groups, Lot A and Lot C. The two animals in Lot A and two additional guinea pigs, in Lot B, "were injected under the skin of belly with $\frac{1}{2}$ c.c. of a virulent culture of the tubercle bacillus suspended in water." The animals in Lot C, which had received the protective treatment alone, "were kept to determine the effects of the attenuated culture." When the guinea-pigs were killed after six weeks, these results appeared:

Lot C. (simply subjected to protective treatment).—Both guinea-pigs present a small ulceration where the attenuated culture has been injected; in the first animal the spleen is a little enlarged and two grey tubercles are visible in the right lung; in the second animal all the organs are perfectly normal.

Lot B. Controls.—Both animals are markedly tubercular.

Lot A.—Both animals are profoundly tubercular, perhaps a trifle more so than the controls (p. 567).

Trudeau repeated this experiment two more times, using different cultures of the same attenuated bacilli—"surface cultures of the attenuated bacillus grown on glycerine-peptone-agar, instead of liquid culture" and "a fresh surface culture of the attenuated bacillus grown at a constant temperature of 37 degrees C."

He concluded from these experiments that

preventive inoculation of the non-living chemical products of the life history of the tubercle bacillus failed . . . to afford any protection against subsequent infection with virulent living tubercle bacilli.

Preventive inoculation with an attenuated but living germ . . . failed to protect against subsequent inoculations with virulent tubercle bacilli. No immunity seems to have been conferred by saturation of the system, which the chemical substances evolved by the microbes during their growth in artificial culture media, or by the production of a mild form of the disease (pp. 567–68).

Though his results were negative, Trudeau expressed optimism

It must not be forgotten, however, that the methods of preventive inoculation which have formed the groundwork of this study are merely tentative and in a field in which we can as yet but grope our way. They may seem crude even now, and in the light of our rapidly advancing knowledge on this subject they will soon appear even more so than at present. Nevertheless, merely as a biological study of the tubercle bacillus these observations seem perhaps worthy of record, and we may, in spite of the improving evidence which they have brought forth, turn to the brilliant announcements recently published with a strong hope that the resources of foreign laboratories or the individual efforts of some earnest worker are about to solve the problem of protective inoculation for this disease, even if the genius of Koch, reaching out along new lines, has not already succeeded in producing a specific treatment for the cure of tuberculosis (Trudeau, 1890, p. 568).

TUBERCULIN ANNOUNCED AS A CURE

This optimism reflected the dramatic announcement of Robert Koch at the International Medical Congress in Berlin, August 4–9, 1890. Though bacteriology had provided minimal therapeutic value so far, it had been important for diagnosis and prophylaxis. Shrady reported on Koch's address. With regard to tuberculosis,

we were on the eve of practical therapeutic developments based upon this science. It was not his custom to publish his investigations until they were completed, but he would make an exception this time. He had not only succeeded in conferring upon guinea-pigs . . . perfect immunity against that disease, but had also discovered means of arresting the growth and multiplication of tubercle bacilli after inoculation (*Medical Record,* vol. 38, no. 6, August 9, 1890, p. 159).

This news created unbounded excitement in the medical world and was broadcast in the popular press. If it was true that a disease that killed one of seven people could be successfully prevented and effectively treated, then bacteriology and immunology had again produced miraculous results.

In October, Shrady put into his "News of the Week" column a direct quote from Koch:

I have at last hit upon a substance which has the power of preventing the growth of tubercle bacilli, not only in a test-tube, but in the body of an animal . . . my researches on this substance . . . are not yet completed, and I can only say this much about them, that guinea-pigs . . . if exposed to the influence of this substance, cease to react to the inoculation of the tuberculous virus, and that in guinea-pigs suffering from general tuberculosis, even to a high degree, the morbid process can be brought completely to a standstill, without the body being in any way injuriously affected. From these researches, I, in the meantime, do not draw any further conclusions than that the possibility of rendering pathogenic bacteria in the living body harmless without injury to the latter, which has hither to been justly doubted, has been thereby established (*Medical Record,* vol. 38, no. 5, October 11, 1890, p. 413).

In the same column it was reported that Dr. Grancher of France "has obtained by cultivation a fluid with which he vaccinates animals and thereby prevents also the subsequent development of tuberculosis" (p. 413). Trudeau published his negative results on immunity in November. He must have read the positive reports by Koch and Grancher and wondered what tricks they had used to get such good results. It is to his credit that, as hope and enthusiasm was building in the medical profession for the Koch cure, he published negative results.

Shrady wrote an editorial aimed at tempering the enthusiasm. He argued that because the remedy was a germicide that destroyed the "vitality or power of growth of the tubercle bacilli" it had limited usefulness. Once lung tissue has been invaded by the phthisical process, "germicides cannot cure phthisis in its secondary and tertiary stages. It remains to be seen, therefore, whether Koch has really supplied us anything which will carry the treatment of tuberculosis any further than it already has been brought" (*Medical Record,* vol. 38, no. 19, November 15, 1890, p. 548). As for prevention, Shrady felt it was already possible if appropriate public health precautions were taken.

Nevertheless, excitement over Koch's announcement was so great that Shrady sent a special correspondent to Berlin to get the latest results from Koch's lab. The correspondent was a former student of Koch who would be working in the lab (*Medical Record,* vol. 38, no. 21, November 22, 1890, p. 580). In an editorial Shrady said, "news during the past week regarding Koch's cure for tuberculosis has in the main confirmed our predictions as to its nature . . . we can only repeat what Koch himself admits, that it can cure the first stages of phthisis only" (p. 579). He reported that Koch had proposed that his remedy be called "parataloid" but that its composition was still secret. Apparently parataloid had an extraordinary selective action, which picked out the tubercular tissue. "The imagination cannot fail to be impressed by the possibilities in therapeutics apparently opened up by Koch. If his discovery turns out to be all that he hopes, the impulse to further research will be immense" (p. 579).

In the next issue Shrady reported that opinions on Koch's discovery were mostly cautious. There seemed to be agreement that it could benefit cases of external tuberculosis, but there was less certainty about its effect on tuberculosis of the lungs (*Medical Record,* vol. 38, no. 22, November 29, 1890, pp. 610–11). He reported that preparation of Koch's lymph was "proceeding rapidly but the quantity required for hospitals and medical associations cannot be made before the end of January" (p. 610). Shrady warned against fraudulent imitators. As Koch had not revealed the composition of his remedy or the method of preparation, the supply was only available from Berlin and there was a suggestion that the German government was trying to control the market.

In the following issue Shrady described the appearance and administration of Koch's lymph as well as the reaction to the injections:

No reaction appears locally [at the injection site] but at the end of four hours severe constitutional effects are manifest in the appearance of rigors with malaise, followed by a temperature which may reach 106 degrees F., with a corresponding increase in the pulse beat from 120 to 160. Sometimes vomiting or prostration or severe dyspnea requiring use of stimulants. When the tuberculous deposit is superficial there is in and around it great tumefaction. The amount of constitutional reaction is said to be governed by the extent of the tubercular deposit (*Medical Record,* vol. 38, no. 23, December 6, 1980, pp. 639–40).

These constitutional effects were short-lived. When injections caused no reaction and scabs that had formed over tubercular swellings left "healthy granulating surfaces," cases were designated as cured. Shrady's correspondent sent a cable from Berlin, dated December 4. Several American physicians had arrived in Berlin to learn about Koch's method—Drs. Ernst of Boston; Abbot of Baltimore; H. P. Loomis, Lindsley, Einhorn, and Stearns of New York; and von Ruck of North Carolina. The correspondent commented on the demonstrations being made of the use of Koch's lymph and emphasized the tentativeness of results at this stage. He advised physicians to wait three or four months for more knowledge to accumulate. The treatments seemed to be used partly in a diagnostic manner (as they produce a reaction in tubercular patients), partly as a curative (but this seemed more uncertain), and partly as a preventive (*Medical Record,* vol. 38, no. 23, December 6, 1980, pp. 637–39). Another report from the Berlin correspondent mentioned that Koch's treatment had been used on people with tubercular bones, glands, and other external tubercular signs. He speculated that the injection supposedly contained no germs, but was a product resulting from "changes produced in the nutrient material by the germs. The remarkable fact is, that the material does not kill the bacilli, as Koch himself expected it would do. The tubercle containing tissue is separated from the healthy tissue, and yet in the former are the living bacilli" (*Medical Record,* vol. 38, no. 23, December 6, 1890, p. 639). The excitement over Koch's discovery continued. Shrady reported that the Paris correspondent had written that Koch's discovery of an alleged "consumption cure" was all that was in the news, and the first trials had begun.

A limited supply of the Koch lymph arrived in New York and was used on twenty cases. Several physicians including Trudeau and Shrady had observed the injections. Little or no reaction was observed, except some rise in temperature, which was much less dramatic than that observed in Berlin. Shrady reported that the lymph was only being used on hospital patients, and the results were being watched by many. "There need be no fear that the Koch method of treating tuberculous afflictions will now have a fair and impartial trial under the care of competent observers, and that perfectly impartial reports will be made" (*Medical Record,* vol. 38, no. 24, December 13, 1890, p. 669). He commented on the confidence of the medical community in Koch, demonstrated by the fact that they had so willingly and eagerly taken up this remedy despite the deplorable fact that its composition was being kept secret. He stated that it would be several months at least before anything about the value of the substance in terms of cure could be determined.

Another physician, Dr. C. Graete from Sanduskey, Ohio, wrote Shrady from Berlin, remarking on the crowds of patients and physicians at the hospitals and clinics where Koch's remedy was being used. He speculated on the composition of the lymph and reported on a number of cases he had observed. They showed the usual constitutional effects from the injections, especially rise in temperature. Four cases of advanced phthisis had postmortems that revealed nothing special on examination of the lungs. But in eight cases in the incipient stages of phthisis, patients treated daily for between fifteen and fifty-six days had relief from night sweats, less cough, and weight gain; and the bacilli could not longer be detected in their sputum (*Medical Record,* vol. 38, no. 24, December 13, 1890, pp. 682–83). Demonstration that the bacilli had disappeared from the sputum was strong evidence in favor of Koch's method.

In the next issue, Shrady emphasized the encouraging but still very tentative results from clinical tests of Koch's lymph. He called for diligence "in the collection of data which shall enable us in due time to form strictly logical conclusions. Hence we are attentively observant and reasonably noncommittal . . . Koch himself, with becoming modesty, claims very little as yet." Shrady deplored the fact "that we are still in the dark as to the actual composition of the fluid for which such wonderful properties are claimed" (*Medical Record,* vol. 38, no. 25, December 20, 1890, p. 699). He sounded a note of caution, quoting a Dr. Bergmann, who said, "There have been no patients cured yet." "In advanced cases of phthisis, it's reported that the disease continues its course despite inoculations. In earlier stages there is apparent improvement, but it is unknown whether it is a cure. Bacilli may remain (*Medical Record,* vol. 38, no. 25, December 20, 1890, pp. 712–13).

The next issue of the *Medical Record* contained a long article by Dr. H. P. Loomis, who reported on his visit to Berlin to obtain a supply of Koch's lymph for Bellevue Hospital. The article described how to obtain the fluid, its appearance, how to prepare it for administration, recommended dosages, the reactions of patients to injections, and its therapeutic value. Expressing caution about its use in the advanced stages of tuberculosis, Loomis was uncertain about the specific action of the injections and whether they reduced the number of bacilli in the sputum. The amount of sputum was first increased, then decreased; night sweats were stopped; and though patients said they felt better, he believed it was too early to take this seriously. "I believe it to be as great a medical discovery as that made by Jenner; that it opens up a hitherto unknown field in the treatment of disease" (Loomis, 1890, pp. 721–24).

At the beginning of 1891 the enthusiasm for Koch's lymph was strong. As the composition was unknown and quantities were limited, this positive response was based upon a few cases observed by physicians who respected Koch's work and desperately wanted a cure for this major killer called tuberculosis. As the supply became more plentiful, many articles and letters reporting experience with Koch's lymph began to appear (*Medical Record,* vol. 39, no. 2, p. 59, pp. 51–52; no. 8, p. 238; no. 11, p. 321; no. 19, p. 545; no. 23, p. 654). Also, those physicians who had viewed its use in Berlin shared their observations (*Medical Record,* vol. 39, no. 1, pp. 27–28; no. 2, pp. 44–47, p. 47, p. 59). Negative reports began to come in. Though not condemning it outright, the medical community in Vienna reported they had not found the remedy to be reliable either in the diagnosis of tuberculosis or in treatment (*Medical Record,* vol. 39, no. 2, January 10, 1891, p. 66).

In February, Koch (1891) revealed the method for preparing the tuberculin. The remedy consisted of a "glycerine extract of the tubercle bacilli." It should be administered subcutaneously with a clean syringe. The most suitable sight is the skin at the back between the shoulder blades and the lumbar region. About five hours after injection the patient becomes violently ill with a temperature of 105.8 degrees F. lasting twelve to fifteen hours. Then the patient feels comparatively well. In the course of three weeks rapidly increasing doses can be given, up to 500 times the original amount. When the point is reached that the reaction is as feeble as that of a nontuberculous patient, it may be assumed that all tuberculous tissue is destroyed. Koch suggested that his remedy made tuberculous tissue necrotic (kills the tissue) and acted only on the living tissue.

With the method clearly described, numerous attempts were made to test Koch's remedy in the following year, and reports were mixed. Sir Joseph Lister returned from Berlin and spoke at King's College Hospital in London. "His impressions were favorable to the remedy. He regarded its action on tubercular disease as simply astounding, both as a curative and a diagnostic agent" (*Medical Record*, vol. 39, no. 4, January 24, 1891, p. 120). Shrady reported the conclusions of Dr. Browicz of Korakow, who rejected the idea that tuberculous tissue became necrotic. He argued that the remedy produced an inflammation of the tissue, which was then carried away with the exudation of this process. Shrady warned that the expulsion of tubercle bacilli could spread them to the lungs and intestines (*Medical Record*, vol. 39, no. 7, February 14, 1891, pp. 209–10; also no. 9, p. 267). Word came from London that "Clinical observers also are finding the ultimate results of the treatment to be far from satisfactory" (*Medical Record*, vol. 39, no. 8, February 21, 1891, p. 243). The quality of parataloid was questioned by a physician who noted that a patient who had been tolerating increasing doses suddenly had a violent reaction when a dose was given from a new batch (*Medical Record*, vol. 39, no. 8, February 21, 1891, p. 247). Sentiment began to develop that Koch's remedy was useful only in incipient cases of tuberculosis (*Medical Record*, vol. 39, no. 11, March 14, 1891, pp. 328–29). A report from Presbyterian Hospital in Chicago noted, "In cases of pulmonary tuberculosis of any considerable standing, there has been no appreciable improvement" (*Medical Record*, vol. 39, no. 12, March 21, 1891, p. 350). And in some circles the sentiment was critical, labeling Koch's remedy as "harmful or, at best does not live up to expectations" (*Medical Record*, vol. 39, no. 19, May 9, 1891, p. 549).

More evidence accumulated. Shrady reported the conclusions of Dr. Detweiler of Falkenstein after four months of using tuberculin on the patients at his sanitorium. Comparing 128 patients who received tuberculin and the climatic cure with fifteen previous years of patients, he concluded that tuberculin's action was different from other remedies but that one cannot predict whether the effect will be good or bad. It should only be used in small doses. It was not a true specific because "it did not render the lung immune or kill the bacilli." It was not yet possible to render a final judgment (*Medical Record*, vol. 39, no. 21, May 16, 1891, p. 575).

At the stated meeting of the New York Academy of Medicine on May 7, 1891, a symposium of clinicians including Trudeau gave their "Observations on the Use of Koch's Tuberculin in the Treatment of Pulmonary Tuberculosis" (*Transactions of the New York Academy of Medicine*, 8:145–67, 1892). From St. Luke's Hospital, Dr. F. D. Kinnicutt reported on forty-two patients he had treated since December 10 and concluded,

It is my distinct impression that tuberculin is capable, in the early stage of pulmonary tuberculosis, of effecting a greater degree of improvement in the physical condition of the lung, and, in more advanced disease, in many of the accompanying symptoms, than has been observed under any other method of purely medical treatment. Its sphere of greatest usefulness will probably be found in its combination with other methods of treatment" (p. 147).

This application of tuberculin was confounded because no controls were used for comparison to the forty-two treated patients. Was the reputed success of tuberculin due to tuberculin itself or to the "other methods of treatment" already being used on the patients?

Dr. Alfred L. Loomis presented thirteen cases of pulmonary tuberculosis that had been treated at Bellevue Hospital from December 18, 1890 to March 11, 1891. He concluded:

While in the majority of our cases an arrest of the tubercular processes has followed the use of the tuberculin, sufficient time has not elapsed to venture an opinion as to the permanence of such arrest. . . . In a minority of our cases the use of the tuberculin has been followed by great activity in the original tubercular areas and a rapid development of new areas. In two instances its use was followed by signs of acute general tubercular infection, which rapidly precipitated a fatal issue. . . . While the expectations of Prof. Koch may not be realized, I believe that after this agent has passed through the siftings of careful and experienced clinicians it will take a permanent place among the aids for the cure of pulmonary tuberculosis (p. 151).

Dr. H. N. Heineman reported on twenty-two cases of pulmonary phthisis with generally negative results. Dr. E. L. Trudeau described eight cases treated since January at the Adirondack Cottage Sanitarium: "by injections of tuberculin combined with all other climatic, hygienic, and therapeutic measures which experience has shown capable of favorably influencing the course of pulmonary phthisis, and even, in some instances of curing the disease" (p. 163). Trudeau detailed these other methods very explicitly, not only to educate but perhaps to impress his colleagues. New York City was the greatest source for both private and sanitarium patients and for financial support.

The measures referred to consisted of a residence in the invigorating climate of the Adirondacks; a systematic, restful out-of-door life, eight to ten hours being spent daily in short walks or sitting on sheltered verandas out-of-doors irrespective of temperature or weather; dry friction to the skin; careful feeding, milk entering largely as an element in the diet; the administration of creosote in doses varying from ten to fifteen drops daily, according to the state of the patient's digestive powers—this being, with slight variations, the usual treatment resorted to in the institution. In addition, in six of the cases, lung expansion in the pneumatic cabinet, with daily inhalations of peroxide of hydrogen according to the plan suggested by Dr. Quimby, were given with a view of producing favorable influence on both the capillary and lymphatic pulmonary circulation. . . . The injections of tuberculin were made generally twice a week, the dose being regulated as to produce as slight a reaction as possible. In cases where the reactions became marked or the patient's nutritive powers showed any sign of depreciation, the intervals between the injections were lengthened and the doses diminished. The amount injected was, however, very slowly but steadily increased until doses of from eighteen to a hundred milligrams were given without any appreciable disturbance (pp. 163–64).

For the eight cases, Trudeau reported "one apparently cured, four greatly improved and still improving, two unimproved, one apparently injured by the treatment. . . . These results, though the number of cases is limited, are encouraging, and were possibly more rapidly obtained than could have been expected by climatic and hygienic measures alone" (p. 165). We can only assume that Trudeau kept a separate record of these cases in his lab. According to the sanitorium case records, only seven cases had started treatment before May of 1891; the results were one cured, two arrested, one unimproved, and three with no discharge data. It is likely that the clinical judgments of success were quite subjective, as no clearly defined criteria had yet been established. Trudeau cautioned his colleagues:

Treatment by injections of tuberculin is not applicable to all cases of phthisis, and in unsuitable cases (and even in apparently favorable cases when rapidly pushed) undoubtedly greatly aggravates the disease and hastens the inevitable end. The decision as to its applicability to a given case depends not only on the amount of disease present, but on its type, and, above all, on the state of the patient's nutritive powers. If these are fair or susceptible of being stimulated, and the pulmonary involvement is not excessive and apparently uncomplicated, injections of tuberculin may be resorted to with a reasonable hope of producing a marked, though possibly, only temporary improvement.
    Koch's method is certainly the first thus far proposed which can be shown by clinical observation to produce a distinct and appreciable impression on the areas of diseased tissue, and the physical signs noted at the bedside support Koch's assumption as to the specific action which tuberculin produces on pulmonary infiltrations of a tubercular nature. It is yet too early to reach any conclusion as to the possibility of obtaining a cure as a result of this specific action, or to predict the remote dangers it may threaten. Tuberculin has no germicidal properties and it does not seem at all probable that it can produce in the individual any immunity against further infection; so that it is only through its specific impression on tubercle, and on account of the marked alteration in the biological relations of the tubercle bacillus to the surrounding tissue which it produces, that a cure may be hoped for (p. 166).

Trudeau then questioned Koch's claims:

The scope of Koch's method of treatment, its evident dangers and its limitations, seem to me to depend greatly upon the fulfillment of its promise of producing immunity. . . .
    Koch himself evidently thought it capable of conferring at least a temporary protection against secondary germ invasion, for he states that "while under its influence guinea-pigs cease to react to tubercular inoculation," and he also says "Meanwhile we must protect the healthy tissues from a fresh invasion of the germs by repeated injections of the remedy." . . .
    My own attempts at the production of artificial immunity in animals by preventive inoculation of tubercular products [1890c] have proved so uniformly unsuccessful that

I am inclined to think the deficiency in Koch's method lies in this very direction, and that injections of tuberculin are powerless to confer immunity (p. 166).

Finally, he advertised his general sanitarium treatment:

The only immunity, therefore, we can invoke to protect the patient against the dangers of reinfection while attempting to bring about, by injections of tuberculin, pathological changes tending to necrosis of tubercle, is that produced by all measures which have been found to improve nutrition. These measures consist of climate, an open-air life, hygiene, feeding, and medical supervision; and although, by combining with these the specific impression exercised by tuberculin on tubercle, the treatment of incipient phthisis seems at present to hold out an added promise, its success or failure will still depend in the future, as in the past, on the persistence and thoroughness of our efforts to stimulate nutrition (pp. 166–67).

At this point Trudeau, while not wanting to judge Koch too severely, was not impressed by this new method. His clinical experience and his laboratory results gave him little reason for enthusiasm. The general methods of therapy that he had experienced in his own case and that he used at the sanitarium were still superior. Ironically, the failure of Koch's tuberculin focused additional attention on the alternative, Trudeau's open-air method, increasing its credibility and appeal.

At the AMA meeting in May, Dr. Karl von Ruck of the Winyah Sanitorium at Asheville, North Carolina, said nearly the same thing. On the basis of twenty-six cases treated with tuberculin, he believed it could be used safely and beneficially but said that more experience by many practitioners was needed to determine its value. However, Dr. Osler of Johns Hopkins reported that only five of twenty-four cases treated there had benefited (*Medical Record,* vol. 39, no. 210, May 16, 1891, pp. 578–79). The next week von Ruck's paper appeared in the *Medical Record* (vol. 39, no. 21, May 23, 1891, pp. 589–92). After ten weeks of experience of using small doses that avoid a general reaction, he claimed patients experienced general improvement in symptoms. He emphasized that improvement occurred from the established general treatments involving diet, climate, and rest; but as improvement with Koch's remedy was more rapid, it should therefore be used in conjunction with these other treatments.

Shrady reported a strongly negative opinion expressed by Dr. J. R. Buist of Nashville at the annual meeting of the Tennessee State Medical Society:

Regarding Koch's parataloid as a remedy for consumption, Dr. Buist said the high expectations so recently excited by these inoculations do not seem to be verified. Certainly for advanced stages of phthisis and many other forms of tuberculosis it is unsuited and positively dangerous; and it is not settled whether any benefit can attend its use in the incipient cases (*Medical Record,* vol. 39, no. 20, May 16, 1891, p. 580).

Dr. Buist's opinion was that emphasis on prevention rather than therapeutic measures would be more important and that education of the public, though difficult, would be more effective. One of the strongest condemnations of Koch's remedy came from the Committee of Physicians of the St. Louis Hospital in Paris. Considering thirty-eight cases, the committee stated that in some cases the general reaction was so intensely alarming that death had been imminent. In eight cases congestion of the lungs resulted. There were two cases of hematuria [blood in the urine], four cases of albuminuria [albumin in the urine], and five or six cases of severe cardiac symptoms. Not one case was cured or nearly cured, and there was scarcely any observable improvement. The committee concluded that "they did not feel justified in continuing this method of treatment, except experimentally" (*American Journal of Medical Sciences,* vol. 101, no. 5, May 1891, pp. 530–31). Most of these papers were based on clinical opinion or study of a few cases. No well-controlled studies were reported.

Trudeau described the excitement at this time:

It would be hard to exaggerate the intense excitement that pervaded the little colony of invalids at Saranac Lake when Koch's first announcement of his specific was published in the daily press, and I had all I could do to prevent several of my patients from rushing over to Berlin at once to be cured. Mr. George Cooper offered to send me to Berlin and pay my expenses, but Dr. Prudden, who knew the conditions advised me not to go and I took his advice.

The first tuberculin I received came in a small glass bulb and was sent me by Dr. Osler, who, with his usual generosity, shared with me the first bottle of the priceless fluid he had just received from Germany. This small bulb, which was supposed to contain a liquid capable of giving life to hopeless invalids, was gazed at with deep emotion by many.

I at once began the injections on a few selected cases at the Sanitarium, and watched the results with keenest interest. Koch had not at that time revealed the nature of his specific. Had I but known that the precious fluid was a glycerin extract of the tubercle bacillus, I could have carried out my observations on a much larger scale, for in my laboratory many flasks of liquid cultures of the tubercle bacillus were growing.

The bitter disappointment which within a few months followed the failure of Koch's treatment to bring about the miraculous cures which were expected from it was shown very soon in a widespread and violent condemnation of the remedy (Trudeau, 1915, pp. 212–14).

According to the case records, Trudeau first used Koch's method on December 20, 1890 (case # 287, admitted October 27, 1890). The notes reveal that the paratoloid first came in December from Osler at Johns Hopkins and then from Koch on February 20, 1891. The patient was discharged on May 14, 1891, and listed as "cured," with the word "arrested" crossed out. In 1891 Trudeau used tuberculin on twenty of the eighty patients who came that year and on seventeen of eighty-one patients in 1892. The sanitarium case records are discouragingly brief. Often the record will say "Koch's Method" (case # 287) or "Koch's Liquid" (case # 293) or "since March 3 has had inoculations twice a week, dose gradually increasing each time" (case # 303). In the fall Trudeau used something called "Modification B" (case # 315, October 21, 1891) or "Mod. Tub." (case # 341) and used this until the end of 1891. In February of 1892 he used "Trudeau B" (case # 378), then "Mod. B. Trudeau" (June 10, case # 386); finally, on February 18, 1893, he used "Hunter's B" (case # 445). It appears that he began with very small amounts (.005 mg) a day, increasing to as much as 100 mg or more per day, but this is difficult to read accurately.

From the case records it is possible to tally results of patients treated with Koch's tuberculin or some modification (see Table 9.1). These results are difficult to interpret because the case records are so incomplete. Perhaps Trudeau kept another set of records on the study patients in his laboratory. A malfunctioning thermostat started a fire that destroyed his lab and home while the family was away in 1893. Detailed records of his use of Koch's method do not exist, but Trudeau did present "The Treatment of Experimental Tuberculosis by Koch's Tuberculin. Hunter's Modification and Other Products of the Tubercle Bacillus" at the Association of American Physicians annual meeting on May 24, 1892 (Trudeau, 1892). Trudeau began his paper by noting that Robert Koch had raised the possibility of tuberculin injections to cure tuberculosis but that this had led to disappointment. Koch's results had been obtained on guinea pigs, but they were not confirmed by other researchers before experiments on humans

Table 9.1
Patients Treated with Koch's Tuberculin or Some Modification

Result	1891*		1892	
	n	%	n	%
Cured	3	15	5	29
Improved	2	10	0	0
Arrested	9	45	1	6
Unimproved	1	5	6	35
Died	0	0	2	12
No discharge information	5	25	3	18
Total	20	100	17	100

*Includes the first patient who began treatments December 20, 1890, and was discharged cured. 1891 and 1892 are the years the patients were admitted. In several cases the treatments lasted longer than twelve months.

were started. He suggested that only after positive results from experimental tuberculosis in animals had been demonstrated should experiments on humans take place. Trudeau had participated in the "gigantic human experiment" himself. By May 1892 he had treated at least twelve patients with unspectacular results. It was not surprising that he would call for "more exact and extended knowledge" from animal studies.

The goal of his research was to obtain more definitive evidence

first, as to the curative effect said to be exercised by Koch's tuberculin upon inoculated guinea pigs; second, as to the curative value and dangers in experimental tuberculosis of the modifications of tuberculin proposed by Hunter [and] to demonstrate, by a few simple experiments, in which part of liquid cultures of the tubercle bacillus the remedial element resides—whether in the bacteria-protein of which the bacilli are composed, or in the albumoses and soluble toxines produced in artificial culture-media as the result of their life history (p. 253).

In the first experiment twelve guinea pigs were inoculated with a pure (virulent) culture of tubercle bacilli grown on glycerin serum. Four of these were kept as controls. Within two weeks the remaining eight were given "injections of Koch's crude tuberculin, beginning at one milligram daily and steadily increasing to one cubic centimeter, the intervals being lengthened as the doses become larger" (p. 253). Trudeau experienced difficulty with these injections. Two of the guinea pigs died "within six hours of taking the same dose that they had previously borne without accident." The four controls lived an average of eighty-eight days, and the six treated animals lived an average of 112 days. Upon autopsy Trudeau observed

In the dead controls the pathologic processes are seen to be more advanced the nearer they occur to the inoculation-wound, while in the treated animals the reverse usually holds true.

The controls showed at autopsy cheesy inoculation-wounds, often still open, cheesy inguinal and retroperitoneal glands, enormous spleen riddled with tubercles and cheesy areas, enlarged tuberculous liver, and a moderate number of young tubercles scattered through the lungs. In the test-animals . . . the inoculation spot is healed and covered with hair; the inguinal glands are firm, only slightly enlarged, and rarely cheesy; the spleen is either moderately tuberculous, or it may even be of normal size and appearance; the liver likewise; while the lungs are solid with cheesy tubercles (p. 254).

Trudeau's explanation for these autopsy results was

It is probable . . . that the curative influence of tuberculin is exercised only when tubercle-tissue has once formed. The reparative processes that it incites seem to follow in the track of the disease, but are powerless to anticipate extension to neighboring structures. Habituation to the injection soon takes place. The dose grows rapidly, as the disease, overcome at one point, spreads to another; and by the time the lungs are attacked, anything short of a poisonous amount will no longer bring about the local reaction necessary to cure. The pulmonary disease, therefore, progresses unchecked, and soon results in the animal's death. . . .

It would seem, . . . that injections of tuberculin exercise a marked remedial influence on the tuberculous lesions of the guinea pig, and can cure the primary ones; but contrary to Koch's belief, the injections cannot "protect the tissues from further invasion of the germs," for infection in these animals may spread from one point to another, even while a cure of the primary lesions is being effected by the treatment (p. 254).

In his earlier experiment Trudeau had used an attenuated culture of tubercle bacilli as an injection to see if it gave protection to later inoculation with live bacilli. It had not. In this experiment he first inoculated the guinea pigs with live bacilli, giving them tuberculosis, then used Koch's tuberculin inoculations to see if they prevented spreading of the disease. While it took these animals longer to die, they still had the disease. These results did not confirm the claims of Robert Koch.

During the time Trudeau was producing these negative results on guinea pigs, he was using various forms of tuberculin on humans. By the end of May 1892 he had started to treat twenty-three patients, according to the case records.

Next, Trudeau, following Hunter and Klebs, attempted to eliminate elements from the tuberculin that produced fever and violent reactions. Noting that neither Koch nor Klebs had given enough information to reproduce their results, he turned to the work of Hunter who had prepared a modified tuberculin and described the process "in terms as clear and concise as to invite other investigators to test his conclusions and attempt to throw some additional light on the points he has so admirably studied" (p. 254). Trudeau appeared to be expressing frustration with Koch's and Kleb's studies and their unwillingness to adhere to the canons of science.

Following Hunter's directions, Trudeau produced two substances, Hunter's "B" and "CB." He repeated the preceding experiment on twelve guinea pigs with "C" and twelve with "CB."

The results show an average life of ninety-two days for the controls, one animal still living seven months after inoculation; an average of eighty-nine days for the animals treated with CB; and of one hundred and twenty days for the animals treated with B, of which two are still living seven months after the virulent inoculation. . . .

Two of the animals treated with CB died unusually early, namely sixty-three and seventy-eight days respectively after inoculation. The autopsies showed a marked tendency to early generalization of the disease; emaciation was extreme; there were no very advanced or extensive caseous processes anywhere, but an enormous amount of young tubercle was equally distributed in all the organs.

The duration of life in the animals dying while under treatment with B was considerably above the average of the controls. The autopsies showed practically the same appearances, and the same attempt at repair in the inoculation-wound, glands, and spleen, as in animals dying while under tuberculin treatment.

The two guinea pigs that are still alive (nearly seven months after the virulent inoculation) show healed inoculation-wounds, no enlarged glands, and their weight is a trifle more than at the beginning of the experiment. The dose of modification B has risen to seven cubic centimeters at an injection; the immediate result of which is to throw the animals instantly into tetanic spasms, from which, however, they recover within an hour. They no longer show any marked rise of temperature following the injections (p. 255).

From these experiments Trudeau concluded

1. In Hunter's modifications the curative principle has been retained. This is especially true of modification B.

2. The fever-producing elements have been, to a certain extent, eliminated, but CB may favor rather than hinder the tendency to generalization.

3. Modification B is as efficient and is safer than either CB or crude tuberculin. Thus far my experience with modification B has confirmed this conclusion (p. 255).

If the case records can be trusted, Trudeau used "MOD.TUB." on case # 341 beginning October 20, 1891, for a year with the result that the patient was discharged 7½ pounds heavier on October 23, 1892, with the disease "arrested," and the tubercle bacillus still present in the sputum. "Modification B" was started on case # 354, October 27, 1891, with similar results. It was used on case # 367 beginning in December 1891 and continued until October 1892, with the patient having sputum free of bacilli and being labeled "cured." He then used "Trudeau B" on # 378 for only about a month and a half; the patient became weaker and was discharged unimproved. The statement in the paper was thus based on four cases; # 354 and # 378 had been discharged, while # 341 and # 367 were still at the sanitarium being treated.

Trudeau separated the bacilli from the culture medium in which they had grown. He obtained the culture medium in the following manner:

Liquid cultures of the tubercle bacillus are filtered through hardened filter paper. To this filtrate one per cent. of carbolic acid is added to preserve it, and it is now ready for use. This fluid contains all of the soluble albumoses and toxins, but no bacterio-protein, and nothing that may have been extracted from the bacilli by heat, as in the manipulation for producing Koch's tuberculin (p. 255).

The bacilli on the filter paper are washed and combined with a "50 percent glycerin and water mixture and put into a sterilizer for two hours. The solution is filtered and the filtrate is a true glycerin extract of the tubercle bacillus."

These two solutions were then injected into "several sets of tuberculous guinea pigs." He concluded that they have, apparently, no marked remedial value. From the autopsies, the 50 percent glycerin solution appears to hinder the natural chimiotactic reaction at the inoculation spot or in the injected organ, and thus to favor a general spread of the disease. Injections of the soluble products contained in the culture-medium in which bacilli have developed produce no local suppuration [pus formation], but all of the characteristic reactions of tuberculin (p. 256).

For the next experiment, "rabbits were inoculated in the anterior chamber of the eye" with live bacilli. "One group was kept as controls, while the remaining animals were divided into equal groups and treated with each of the solutions" (p. 256). Those animals injected with the glycerin extract of the tubercle bacillus containing dead bacilli died and no beneficial effect was observed on the eye lesions. The animals injected with the soluble products contained in filtered culture medium showed "no serious deterioration in the animal's general health."

During the first six weeks, the treatment appears to have only sensibly hastened the progress of the disease, but about the seventh week, if the injections were begun within a few days after inoculation, an improvement in the eye-lesions first shows itself. . . . From this time, as the irritation caused by each injection disappears, marked improvement is apparent. The caseous areas slowly melt away, the dilated blood vessels shrink and disappear, intra-ocular pressure diminishes, the cornea clears, and from twelve to eighteen weeks from the beginning of treatment the eye is to all appearances cured, in the sense that it has been restored as nearly to its normal condition as is consistent with the lesions existing when treatment was begun. . . . As to the permanency of this apparent cure time alone can decide. . . . In the few autopsies made on animals whose eyes had been cured, no tuberculous disease was found in other organs (p. 257).

Trudeau concluded

It is, thus, not to the bodies of the bacilli, but to the liquid that they have impregnated with the products of their life-history that we must look for the remedial element contained in ripe cultures. . . . It is to this element of liquid cultures that we must turn in future attempts to separate a substance free from the dangers of tuberculin, and yet capable of exercising, it may be, to a greater or less degree, a curative influence over visceral tuberculosis (p. 257)

While the number of rabbits used in these studies was never mentioned, on the basis of these results Trudeau stated that Koch's tuberculin did not cure experimental tuberculosis in the guinea pig. On the other hand the results on the eyes of rabbits were promising and needed to be followed up.

    At the next meeting of the Association of American Physicians, in 1893, Trudeau had to temper the claim he had made in 1892:

A more extended experience has shown me that the cure of inoculation tuberculosis in the rabbit's eye by this method is by no means always a constant result or one which can be brought about invariably at will. I have failed often where I had every reason to expect success, and I have succeeded where I had no special reason to hope for a favorable result. This inconsistency in results may be explained by the great difficulty of controlling the relation existing between all the factors involved in the problem, such as the virulence of the bacilli injected, their number, the virulence of the microbes from which the tuberculin was made, and the degree of individual resistance possessed by each animal. Cures do occur, however, and appear to have a certain degree of permanence, as the two animals I now show you illustrate (Trudeau, 1893, p. 97).

By displaying the animals, Trudeau could at least demonstrate that he had produced a cure. But he could not produce it consistently so that others could reproduce his work.

At this meeting Trudeau confessed another error he had made in an earlier paper (1890b) to the Association of American Physicians, in 1890, comparing two quite different cultures of the bacillus. He had assumed that the less virulent culture (no. 2) from Dr. Currier in France had been human. From reading the bacteriologists Muffici, Koch, Metchnikoff, Courmont, Dor, and Loeb, he discovered that the weak bacillus was actually "avian tubercle bacillus" and that it "is apparently a race by itself and that it presents quite constant cultural and pathogenic peculiarities not observed in the microbe originally discovered, studied, and described by Koch" (Trudeau, 1893, p. 97). He noted that the avian bacillus was harmless for dogs and guinea pigs but fatal to rabbits. However "when a small amount—0.05 to 0.25—of liquid culture grown a month direct from the chicken is injected under the skin, the animal generally recovers; an abscess is formed at the site of the inoculation which tends slowly to soften and become diffuse, and, finally, if the animal survives, disappears almost entirely" (Trudeau, 1893, p. 98). This suggested to Trudeau the possibility of using avian bacilli for preventive inoculation. He had failed to produce immunity in an earlier experiment (1890), but new research had come out in which

Richet and Herzicourt have . . . claimed to produce complete immunity in dogs by intravenous inoculations of bird tubercle bacilli. These experimenters found that though harmless to the dog when first derived from the chicken, bird bacilli, by long cultivation in liquid media, became pathogenic for this animal, and by thus grading the virulence of the injections complete immunity against any form of tubercular infection was produced in the dog (Trudeau, 1893, p. 98).

Following this example, Trudeau grew cultures from chicken lesions in bouillon for five weeks, then six months. This avian bacillus was injected two times subcutaneously in rabbits in doses of 0.025 and 0.05, twenty-one days apart.

About one in four of the rabbits died within three months, profoundly emaciated, but without any visible tubercular lesions. The remaining animals recovered and were apparently in good health when, together with an equal number of controls, they were inoculated in the anterior chamber of the eye with cultures of Koch's bacillus derived from the tuberculous lesions of the rabbit and cultivated about three months on glycerin-agar (Trudeau, 1893, p. 98).

The controls displayed a very different pattern of reaction than did the rabbits that received the avian-bacilli preventive inoculation. In the controls,

two days after the introduction of the virulent material in the eye little or no irritation is observed, and little is to be noticed for two weeks, when a steadily increasing vascularity manifests itself, small tubercles appear on the iris which gradually coalesce and become cheesy, intense iritis and general inflammation of the structures of the eye develop, the inoculation wound becomes cheesy, and in six to eight weeks the eye is more or less completely destroyed and the inflammation begins to subside. The disease, however, remains generally localized in the eye for many months, and even permanently (Trudeau, 1893, p. 98).

In the vaccinated animals . . . the introduction of the virulent bacilli at once gives rise to a marked degree of irritation. On the second day the vessels of the conjunctiva are tortuous and enlarged, whitish specks of fibrinous-looking exudation appear in the iris and in the anterior chamber, and more or less iritis supervenes, but at the end of the second to the third weeks, when the eyes of the controls begin to show progressive and steadily increasing evidence of inflammatory reaction, the irritation in those of the vaccinated animals begins slowly to subside and the eye to mend . . . until in from six to twelve weeks in successful cases all irritation has disappeared and the eyes present, as in the animals I now show you, but the fibrous evidence of the traumatism and the inflammatory processes which have been set up by the inoculation (Trudeau, 1893, p. 98).

Trudeau admitted that some of these animals slowly relapsed and pointed out "small tubercles growing on the iris" of his display rabbit. Nevertheless, he said he had repeated the experiment "on three sets of rabbits with about the same results each time." He concluded:

The vaccinations as practiced are of themselves, in some instances, fatal, but the fact remains that where recovery takes place a marked degree of immunity has been acquired. I do not lay any claim, therefore, to have produced a complete or permanent immunity by a safe method, but it seems to me that these eyes constitute a scientific demonstration of the fact that in rabbits preventive inoculation of bird tubercle bacilli can retard and even abort an otherwise progressive localized tubercular process so completely as to prevent destruction of the tissues threatened, and that the future study of antitubercular inoculation may not be as entirely hopeless as it has until recently appeared (Trudeau, 1893, p. 98).

As it turned out this optimism was premature. The next year, at the Association of American Physicians meeting in May 1894, Trudeau had to admit failure (evidently the rabbit cages were not destroyed by the fire):

In a morbid process, however, following so irregular a course, and of so relapsing a nature as tuberculosis, time must ever be the crucial test that should be applied to any apparently favorable results obtained, and I therefore report briefly the further results of these experiments.

The curative effects of the tuberculin on the eye-lesions, which, as I showed, may go on apparently to absolute disappearance of the tuberculous process in the eye, is in but very rare instances permanent, and a strong tendency to relapse sooner or later becomes apparent. Even after the eyes have remained free from any morbid manifestation for as long as twelve months, will this tendency to recurrence manifest itself (Trudeau, 1894, pp. 346–47).

He was in good company. All other attempts at the production of artificial immunity to tuberculosis in animals had failed. What he did claim was that he produced "at least a relative degree of artificial immunity." Avian bacilli inoculations had delayed the destruction of the rabbit's eye by as much as twelve months. But the "immunity" was only relative. The process had been temporarily delayed. This was not the result that Trudeau desired, and he dropped this line of animal research.

10

Salvaging Tuberculin

After reporting on eight cases, in May of 1891, at the New York Academy of Medicine, Trudeau gave another report at the ninth annual meeting of the American Climatological Association in June 1892. In this paper he made a subtle change in emphasis. In May 1891 he had investigated whether tuberculin was useful as a vaccine; but as sentiment built against tuberculin, he now asked whether the injections would augment his general method of treatment. "The ideal plan of treatment in tuberculosis would, therefore, be one that would enable us, while improving our patient's general condition, to stamp out this infectious element within his tissues, and thus obtain a more permanent cure" (p. 298).

Trudeau experimented on thirteen patients using Koch's tuberculin for "an average period of eleven months." The results were

6 incipient cases
    3 apparently cured
    2 arrested
    1 improved
4 advanced cases
    2 arrested
    2 failed
3 far-advanced cases
    1 improved
    2 failed

He concluded, "my impression was that in many cases, for a time at least, a distinct and specifically beneficial effect was produced, not so much on the general condition of the patient as on the malady itself; unfortunately, the cases most suitable for this treatment are precisely those in which recovery may be hoped for under the more tedious but much safer climatic and out-of-door plan, but in at least some of these under observation the cure was apparently hastened by the injections (p. 299).

Trudeau seemed to be hanging on to thin threads of hope. As he had no controls, but was comparing these results to his experience with other presumably similar cases, that was all he had as a basis for such statements. Ultimately he was forced to reject Koch's tuberculin. "Its uncertainty of action and its very evident dangers have seemed to me, however, to outweigh its curative influence, and, until further research has opened the way to safer treatment by this method, our sole dependence must still be placed on a favorable environment, and our best efforts continue to be directed to a thorough application of all measures that improve nutrition" (p. 299).

The second part of his paper discussed ten cases treated with Hunter's Modification B.

4 incipient cases

    4 apparently cured (no bacillus in sputum)

3 advanced cases

    1 arrested

    1 improved

    1 unimproved

3 far-advanced

    1 improved

    2 unimproved

Judging these data, he wrote, "To anyone familiar with the irregular course and relapsing nature of pulmonary tuberculosis it is quite evident that no conclusion of value as to any special treatment for this disease can be reached in a few months, but as far as such a limited experience can prove anything, I have been favorably impressed with the freedom from ordinary complications and with the excellent results produced in so short a time by injections of the modified tuberculin" (p. 300). Trudeau's statements were based on comparing these ten cases with his previous experience. While such subjective judgments are suspect today, in 1892 they carried some credibility. The paper was printed in the *Proceedings of the American Climatological Association,* vol. 9, 1892, pp. 18–23, and in the *Medical News,* vol. 61, 1892, pp. 298–300. In those days peer review of papers presented to meetings and printed in journals did not exist. Members of the American Climatological Association were expected to present papers, which were automatically published. Editors of journals attended these meetings and reprinted those they judged to be worthy. George Gould, editor of the *Medical News*, corresponded with Edward Trudeau quite freely. It was in the fall of 1892 that he sent Trudeau the accusations against him by certain AMA members regarding the consultation clause.

Although he had little interest in the conventional behaviors and social requirements of the American Medical Association, Trudeau was accused of a breach of "medical" ethics, disobeying the "consultation clause" of the AMA, by Dr. Augustus K. Gardner, a stalwart allopathic physician from Washington. A copy of the accusation was sent to Trudeau by Gould. It was a page torn out of the *Medical Mirror* "notes and items":

Mrs. Harrison is evidently week by week losing ground, occasioned by the rapid development of tuberculosis following an attack of grip of a year or two ago. . . . The one thing naturally which I regret is that the case of Mrs. Harrison could not have been under the care of members of the regular profession whose attainments were of such order as to command a national reputation, instead of irregulars, as irregular in this day and age is another name for mediocrity.

How a lawyer with a logical mind like President Harrison could place his loved ones under the care of infinitesimal cranks is beyond my comprehension.

In this connection, that which strikes me at this distance as strange, is the fact that Dr. E. L. Trudeau, an active member of the New York State Medical Association, was for a long time in daily consultation with the two homeopaths in charge of the case. This is a problem in ethics which I beg leave most respectfully to refer to those stalwart defenders of the faith.

Commenting upon Gardner, Gould wrote Trudeau,

I have received quite a number of letters lately . . . in reference to the matter bespoken in this wretched sheet, of which I send you a page enclosed. You will understand of course, that I speak of it only because I thought you might like to know how many feel about it. My answer to the letters is simply that I have nothing to do with it. . . . Copies of Washington daily papers have been sent to me containing column-long interviews by this Dr. Gardner, who it seems has made the greatest advertising use possible out of the case. Very sincerely your friend. Geo M. Gould, November 3, 1892.

On the back of Gould's letter is what appears to be a draft of Trudeau's reply:

Let me thank you for drawing my attention to the disparaging things which are said of me in the papers on account of my connections with Mrs. Harrison's case. I have no answer to make in print to such attacks. To you however, I will merely say that I have never either written for publication or spoken to reporters *a single word* in regard to this case whatever Dr. Gardner may have seen fit to make me say. I went to see Mrs. Harrison first at the President's urgent request—To refuse my aid in a remote region like this to a woman suffering from intense dysponea [labored or difficult breathing] (and which I could and did relieve by aspiration [removal of fluids from the lung cavity]) because her physician was a homeopath would in my opinion be inhuman bigotry. After this I rendered what assistance I could in urging the advisability and safety of a speedy removal to Washington and took the responsibility of the move upon myself—If such acts are regarded by others as criminal I am certainly guilty and as I cannot see that I have any regress and feel I have done nothing to be ashamed of I must be content to remain silent. You may however, if you care to tell any of your correspondents that I am not a member of the New York State Medical Association, and that body is not therefore to blame for my shortcomings. Sincerely, Edward L. Trudeau (Trudeau Institute Archives).

This exchange illustrates Trudeau's primary dedication to caring for patients. The older rules of professional etiquette had been replaced by the criterion of medical knowledge and common courtesy. The "ethics" and politics of his profession were insignificant under such circumstances. Six years before he had become a charter member of the Association of American Physicians, an organization that rebelled against just such ethics and politics practiced by the American Medical Association.

By 1892 Trudeau was a vital participant in the medical debates about pulmonary disease. His clinical experience must have been increasing tremendously. He was seeing eighty patients a year at the sanitarium. For the last decade he had treated numerous summer visitors. The village of Saranac Lake was beginning to develop "cure cottages" for paying guests and call itself the Pioneer Health Resort. He and his proteges in the community saw most of these patients as well. From the tiny lab attached to his house he had produced several animal studies, presented before prestigious medical meetings and published in respected medical journals. Because of his acquaintance with the European and American literature he had developed knowledge and skill in bacteriology and immunology. All of these things made Trudeau stand out above the majority of his colleagues. Because his health condition would not allow him to leave his beloved mountains and woods, he followed his own interests and avoided joining a medical school faculty. In fact, those physicians and students who were "fortunate" to have incipient cases of tuberculosis flocked to the sanitarium as patients and resident assistants because they could continue their education in this close community of seekers. Dr. Walter B. James of New York City described what happened to several of the medical students with tuberculosis that he sent to the sanitarium in the woods

I would send them to Saranac with a letter to him and with advice to put themselves entirely in his hands, for I knew what the result would be; a few weeks or a few months, perhaps even a year, spent on an open porch, later with an electric light over the couch where, presently, medical literature, especially the literature of tuberculosis would be studied; then with the absence of fever and the return, in some measure, of physical vigor, an opportunity to do a few hours or a half day's work in the laboratory, and as the establishment of an interest that would last for the rest of their lives and leave them further advanced in their profession at the end of their cure than they would have been had they pursued their original course of life. Many of the most useful and productive workers in the field of tuberculosis now scattered throughout this country and Canada, are graduates of Saranac, who there, under Trudeau, found health and encouragement to enter upon a life of research. . . . every evening for many, many years in his cozy library there was an informal gathering of the younger and older doctors . . . and the discussion was almost always of matters in some way related to the disease that had brought them there. These gatherings . . . constituted a school in the truest sense. . . . His patience in listening to his pupils, his kindliness and complete absence of arrogance, the freedom with which he gave to everyone all that he knew. These qualities, together with the indefinable charm that drew these young men to him, made him a great teacher (James, 1916, p. 98).

Edwin R. Baldwin was not a student, but he was twenty-eight and had completed medical school. He was admitted December 27, 1892 (case # 458). After his discharge on September 18, 1893, he stayed in Saranac Lake, where he developed his own practice and became a colleague of Dr. Trudeau. Having used his own microscope to detect bacilli in his sputum, Baldwin came to Saranac Lake and was on the waiting list for six weeks before he was admitted to the sanitarium. Trudeau invited him to the lab the day after he came to town, and Baldwin offered to help him.

I was overjoyed to find such a congenial companion. A well educated physician who wanted to work in my laboratory was a find for me indeed; for not only could he help me with the work, but I could discuss my experiments and my problems with him, and this proved to be an unfailing interest to us both. Dr. Baldwin in those days, of course, knew even less than I did about the new science of bacteriology, and I gladly taught him all I knew; and as gladly does he teach me now the latest advances in a branch of medical science in which he is an expert and an acknowledged authority. Many happy hours did we spend working in the laboratory together (Trudeau, 1915, p. 218).

The two men complemented each other in several ways. Trudeau had the ideas, but Baldwin had the organization. One of the first things he did was study the case records of the sanitarium to see what the actual statistical results were. Up until this time Trudeau had not had time for this detail. Baldwin institutionalized the care methodology, making sanitarium life considerably more routine and orderly. For their research, Trudeau read the French and American literature, Baldwin read German and English articles. Between the two of them they could keep up with most of the significant literature in their field (Brown, 1931). Around 1906, when Trudeau's health became very delicate, Baldwin took over the laboratory; he continued its work after Trudeau's death in 1915.

Another young doctor who appeared for the cure was H. M. Thomas in the fall of 1888. Francis Delafield had sent him with a note saying, "He had red hair and both lungs are involved, so I think there is no hope for him. In spite of this gloomy prognosis, based on two such divergent factors, Dr. Thomas recovered his health completely and has practiced medicine in Baltimore and taught neurology at the Johns Hopkins Medical School ever since" (Trudeau, 1915, p. 222). Thomas helped out in the sanitarium and experimented with hydrofluoric acid inhalations until he recovered. The Trudeaus often visited the Thomases on their trips to Baltimore.

In 1904 Dr. J. Woods Price came for the cure and stayed on at Saranac Lake to care for patients in the sanitarium as well as those receiving care in the increasing number of cure cottages multiplying throughout the village.

The Saranac Laboratory was a place where Trudeau could hunt and fish in his invalid condition. It brought him recognition and respect from professional colleagues, introduced him to professional societies, legitimated the rest-and-fresh-air care of his sanitarium, and secured him a following of younger colleagues who carried on his work.

TRAGEDY

In this period the Trudeaus' daughter Chatte had caused them extreme concern. Sent to a girls' school in New York City at the age of sixteen, she came home at Easter of the first year, "pale and listless." Trudeau wrote,

At first her letters and the accounts we received showed us she was homesick and not very happy, but in January she wrote she didn't feel well and our friends said her appetite had fallen off and that she had indigestion. I laid all this to the confinement of school and city life, but as she did not seem to get any better I began to be anxious, and finally wrote to her to come home for Easter and let me take a look at her. I met her at the train and brought her home, and I never shall forget the shock her appearance gave me. From a plump, robust young woman she had changed to a pale, listless girl, and as she went upstairs to see her mother I went into my office and shut the door. The terrible truth flashed upon me as I remembered how my brother appeared when he was taken ill and came to see me in Newport. I knew it was the same old story, and I felt stunned and had to wait a long time to get hold of myself again before joining the family circle. . . . I felt from the first this was the same type of disease my brother had; the type that progresses rapidly and against which treatment is of no avail. . . . For nearly three years we watched helplessly her young life fade away under the relentless attacks of her disease (Trudeau, 1915, pp. 231–33).

Trudeau admitted that his work was an escape from the despair he felt at home. "During these sad years of Chatte's struggle for life my wife and I ever lived with heavy hearts, though we tried to show her only smiling faces. It was easier for me, because I had to work. I had to listen to the daily appeals of the sick. I had to keep the work at the Sanitarium and Laboratory going, and to that extent I could forget" (Trudeau, 1915, p. 233).

Chatte died on March 20, 1893, and a curious set of events combined to bring Trudeau to his knees. "The summer after Chatte's death we spent in our camp at Paul Smith's as usual, and I threw myself unreservedly into the medical work there, at the Sanitarium, and in Saranac Lake. I had not been at all well since Chatte's death. All the summer I was nervous and sleepless, had constant headaches and was tired most of the time; and when we went back to Saranac Lake for the winter I was feeling wretched" (Trudeau, 1915, p. 255). In November the Trudeaus went to New York City:

Our little cottage was closed—all but the laboratory end—and Dr. Baldwin, whose house was across the street, worked there daily and kept the cultures and experiments going while I was away. We stopped in New York at a little apartment hotel, where I got accommodations reasonably, and we were engaged as usual in seeing our friends and enjoying our visit, when one night I was taken suddenly with a violent chill, followed by a very high temperature, and within a few hours I was more acutely ill than I had ever been before. My friend, Dr. Walton, came to see me and called in Dr. Loomis. They got me a nurse, and for a long time the diagnosis was very obscure. I believe they finally decided I had an abscess of the kidney, but it was a painful attack, and although I lived through it I never recovered from it, and it has never ceased to harass and disturb me more or less, so that I have never slept more than an hour or two at a time ever since (Trudeau, 1915, pp. 255–60).

In the same week that he was suffering from this illness the Trudeaus received bad news:

When the nurse opened the door I wondered why Dr. Loomis had left his office at nine o'clock in the morning, but I could see he looked very solemn and I realized something had happened. In an instant the thought flashed through my mind that Ned, who had gone to Yale, was dead. Dr. Loomis had a telegram in his hand, and as he came to my bedside he said, "Trudeau, I have bad news for you. Dr. Baldwin has just wired me your house was entirely destroyed by a fire originating from the little lamp in the Laboratory; very little was saved." I had expected to hear that Ned was dead, and the news was rather a relief than a shock. I said, "I am so glad that is all. We can get another house" (Trudeau, 1915, p. 256).

The illness continued to bother Trudeau for the next twenty-two years of his life.

The fire produced a response that must have been a tremendous encouragement to Dr. and Mrs. Trudeau.

As soon as I was well enough to see anyone, Mr. Cooper came to see me. After talking a little while he looked embarrassed and said: "I am sorry about the Laboratory and the house, and I want to do something about it. You have no house to go to when you return. I have a lease of the cottage opposite your house; just as soon as you are well enough to go back you can have that cottage for as long a time as you want it. As to the laboratory, I want you to begin to plan a good stone and steel laboratory; one that will never burn up. Plan it just as you want it, complete, and I will be glad to pay for it and give it to you personally" (Trudeau, 1915, pp. 258–59).

Dr. Hodenpyl brought him a new microscope, a gift from himself, Prudden, and others at the Physicians and Surgeons Laboratory. Dr. William Osler wrote Trudeau a very encouraging letter. Other friends expressed their concern and support. George Cooper's sisters were examples.

The Cooper carriage was at our disposal, and my wife got some fresh air in this way. The Misses Cooper made us promise that just as soon as I could be moved we should all be taken to their beautiful house on Twenty-first Street, so my wife and I, with Francis and his nurse, were soon established in most luxurious quarters in Gramercy Park. . . . No friends could have done more than they did to nurse me back to life, and as soon as I was able to travel, which was quite late in December, we all returned to Saranac Lake and occupied the Cooper cottage (Trudeau, 1915, pp. 259–60).

Emeline Cooper had been admitted to the sanitarium March 28, 1892, treated for more than a year, and discharged "cured" on September 12, 1893 (case # 386). It is doubtful that she fit the criteria of patients with financial need, but the Coopers were good friends.

Another boost to Trudeau's morale came when he had to negotiate with the fire insurance company. The house had been insured, but at first

the agent called on me and told me I had entirely forfeited my insurance, first by leaving the house untenanted without permission, and also by leaving a kerosene lamp burning there constantly when no one was in the house. This I expected; and I was much surprised when he added that all over the country my loss had become known, and that much indignation had been shown when it was given out that the insurance companies considered the insurance forfeited, and much sympathy was expressed. He said the insurance companies had decided they would pay my insurance, provided I would write them a note they could publish stating that they had treated me most liberally. This I was very glad to do, and they paid every cent, which was a great help toward building the new house (Trudeau, 1915, pp. 260–61).

This must have been a great load off Trudeau's shoulders. Whether his friends in high places pressured the insurance company will never be known. The sanitarium was not a source of income and not intended to be. Trudeau was financially comfortable. The private patients sent by Dr. Loomis and others in his circle of professional colleagues provided a comfortable income and a reservoir of wealthy donors ready to support his work. Ironically, Trudeau probably cared for a larger group of families with wealth in the Adirondacks than he would have encountered in Manhattan. The mountains attracted an elite segment of people from large urban centers like Philadelphia, Boston, and New

York who were wealthy enough to summer in hotels or to own private camps. Had he stayed in Manhattan, Trudeau's practice would have been limited to that city.

The new house was completed in the fall of 1894, and the laboratory was finished that winter. It was the first lab in the country dedicated to the study and cure of tuberculosis. Both still stand on Church Street in Saranac Lake. The library of the laboratory was given by Horatio Garrett of Baltimore, and the research was supported by George Cooper and his sister, John Garrett, and Mrs. A. A. Anderson, among others (Trudeau, 1903, p. 133). With the help of Dr. Baldwin and capable residents at the sanitarium, Trudeau produced a new set of publications.

THE SEARCH FOR IMMUNITY

After the addition of Baldwin to the staff, Trudeau gained not only a skilled physician but also an interested lab partner. One of the first publications produced in the new Saranac Laboratory was an investigation of the claims of the German bacteriologist, Edwin Klebs.

Klebs, having observed that tubercle bacilli in cultures die when a certain period in their culture is reached, holds that they perish because they produce toward the end of their existence in the culture medium a peculiar germicidal substance which destroys them; that by the chemical processes he describes, he has obtained this specific substance freed from the poisonous alkaloids and albumoses also produced by the microbes during their growth, and present in tuberculin; that he has succeeded in separating from over-ripe cultures this germicidal substance, which he calls "sozalbumose," and that it is the natural specific for this dreaded disease (Trudeau, 1895, p. 872).

Trudeau and Baldwin, following Klebs's directions carefully, prepared large quantities of what Klebs called "antiphthisin," by collecting the fluid filtered from the overripe bouillon cultures of tubercle bacilli. Trudeau had used a similar substance before (Trudeau, 1890). Using various reagents, the antiphthisin was subjected to a qualitative analysis and determined to consist of "an albumose, or peptone-like body" that had been produced by the bacilli. After inoculating guinea pigs with antiphthisin they concluded: "The effects of large doses of 'antiphthisin' were similar in all respects to those produced by small doses of tuberculin" (p. 873).

Next they mixed a suspension of a virulent culture of tubercle bacilli with 3 cc of pure "antiphthisin," let it stand for an hour, and injected five guinea pigs with it. These animals and controls injected with the virulent culture all died. In fact, the experimental animals died an average of eleven days sooner than the controls. They concluded "Antiphthisin possesses, under the conditions stated above, no germicidal power on the tubercle bacillus which can be demonstrated in vitreo" (p. 874). As they had shown that Kleb's "antiphthisin" could not kill the tubercle bacillus, the next question became, could it produce immunity by inoculation? Twelve guinea pigs were inoculated with virulent bacilli. Six were kept as controls, and the other six were injected the following day with "0.25 c.c. 'antiphthisin' one-tenth conc." These injections were continued and increased, so that after a month they were receiving "1.5 c.c. 'antiphthisin.' " The dose was reduced to 1 cc every two or three days until death. "The average duration of life for the control animals was thirty-nine days, for the treated, thirty-three days. A similar experiment was made with 'tuberculocidin' [another Klebs product] purchased in open market, with materially the same results" (p. 873). Trudeau and Baldwin concluded: "When applied to animals . . . neither 'tuberculocidin' nor 'antiphthisin' had any curative influence over the course of experimental tuberculosis in the guinea pig" (p. 874). Finally, they investigated why bacilli in overripe cultures were destroyed. "Dr. Kleb's observation that if a culture medium in which tubercle bacilli have once developed be replanted no growth will occur, was several times confirmed by us. In testing carefully, however, such a medium before planting, and after the germs have ceased to develop on it, it was observed that its reaction had become markedly changed. . . . After an abundant crop of the bacilli has developed on its surface it may be noticed that its reaction has become more or less markedly acid" (p. 873).

They concluded: "Since cultures of the tubercle bacillus become acid as they grow, . . . it may be inferred that the limitation of the growth of the tubercle bacillus in such a culture medium is most likely due to the acidity induced in the medium, rather than to any specific germicidal substance produced therein" (p. 874). This paper effectively destroyed Klebs's claims. For Trudeau to question the work of a reputable European bacteriologist certainly gained him stature among Americans, and (sadly, for other reasons) probably among the French as well.

TUBERCULIN AS A DIAGNOSTIC AGENT

By 1895 the European and American enthusiasm for Koch's tuberculin had shifted to condemnation of its properties as a specific germicide, a therapeutic agent, and a vaccine. Trudeau, however, had continued to use it sparingly. Impressed by some European bacteriologists who discovered that tuberculin could be used in the diagnosis of tuberculosis, he described fourteen cases of suspected tuberculosis in which the diagnosis could not be made "by ordinary means" (Trudeau, 1897a). After injection with as much as three milligrams of tuberculin, seven produced the typical rise in temperature (illustrated in the paper by a twenty-one-day temperature chart). Of these seven, six "have shown at sometime or other, clinical evidence of pulmonary tuberculosis" and one "has been lost sight of and reported dead." Of the seven cases that did not show a reaction to the tuberculin, "two of the patients have passed from under observation, but the others have remained well thus far."

Trudeau suggested rules for giving the "tuberculin test" in a standardized and objective way.

The range of the patient's temperature is ascertained by taking it at 8 A.M., 3 P.M., and 8 P.M. for three or four days before making the test. The first injection should not exceed five milligrams, and if any fever is habitually present should be even less, and is best given early in the morning or late at night as the typical reaction usually begins, in my experience, within six or twelve hours. Such a small dose, while it will often be sufficient to produce the looked-for rise of temperature, has under my observation never produced unpleasant or violent symptoms. An interval of two or three days should be allowed between each of the two or three subsequent injections it may be necessary to give, as reaction in very rare cases may be delayed for twenty-four or even thirty-six hours. On the third day a second dose of one milligram is given, and if no effect is produced, a third of two milligrams three days later. In the great majority of cases of latent tuberculosis an appreciable reaction will be produced by the time a dose of two milligrams has been reached. If no effect has been caused by the tests applied as above I have usually gone no further, and concluded that no tuberculous process was present, or at least not to a degree which need be taken into account in advising the patient on which would warrant insisting on a radical change in his surroundings and mode of life. If some slight symptoms, however, have been produced by a dose of two milligrams, it may be necessary to give a fourth injection of three milligrams in order to reach a positive conclusion. Nevertheless, it should be borne in mind that in a few cases the exhibitions of even larger doses may cause reaction and indicate the existence of some slight latent tuberculous lesion, and the test should not, when applied within the moderate doses described, be considered absolutely infallible (Trudeau, 1897a, p. 690).

In the same month, May 1897, Dr. James Whittaker gave a paper to the Association of American Physicians in which he presented similar results. Both of these papers were replications of European studies and confirmed tuberculin's value in the early diagnosis of tuberculosis, even before bacilli appeared in the sputum. Trudeau still argued that the diagnosis of incipient disease could "generally be made by a careful consideration of the history of the case, the rational symptoms, and the physical signs collectively, aided by microscopic examination of any expectoration obtainable from the patient" (Trudeau, 1897a, p. 687). When this usual procedure failed, the tuberculin test could be used. This was especially valuable, as all of Trudeau's clinical experience had shown that the earlier one started treating tuberculosis, the greater was the probability of recovery.

CONTINUED SEARCH FOR ARTIFICIAL IMMUNITY

Trudeau could not give up the hope that he might create artificial immunity. He had been trying to do this since 1890 (Trudeau 1890c, 1892b, 1893,

1894), with disappointing results. After Dr. de Schweinitz claimed to produce immunity in guinea pigs by using living attenuated cultures originally obtained from the Saranac Laboratory, Trudeau tried again (1897b). He had noticed that these particular bacilli, which had been cultured since 1891, had become attenuated.

I began to notice after two years cultivation that a great majority of the guinea-pigs inoculated with this culture lived for many months beyond the usual time, and the virulence of the germ was evidently decreasing. It was not, however, before 1894, that I observed that many of these animals recovered completely from the inoculation, while a few still died of chronic tuberculous lesions. At present, if twenty animals be inoculated with this attenuated germ, which has been grown for six years continuously on artificial media, with perhaps one or two exceptions, all survive and ultimately recover completely (Trudeau, 1897b, p. 1850).

He was convinced that prolonged cultivation produced an attenuated bacillus that had lost much of its specific pathogenic power. To see whether this attenuated bacillus could produce immunity, Trudeau performed this experiment.

A certain disturbance of health and loss of weight is always caused by the inoculation of this attenuated culture, but the animals after three months seem to have completely recovered. If at this time they are inoculated with virulent bacilli, together with an equal number of controls, the prolongation of life in the vaccinated animals will be apparent in every case. In several lots I have noticed the death of all the controls to occur before a single vaccinated animal had died. Complete immunity, however, has not been attained in my experience so far, by this method, although some of the animals have occasionally lived as long as eighteen months after the virulent inoculation. . . . The immunity caused by this preventive inoculation seems, as far as I have gone to increase . . . with time, but unfortunately I have but a few animals to prove this fact (Trudeau, 1897b, p. 1850).

If he waited long enough the animals eventually died of tuberculosis, but this relative immunity gave him a bit of hope. He concluded:

That such a thing as artificial immunity against tuberculous infection is a possibility seems gradually being demonstrated by these and similar experiments, as the marked prolongation of life in the vaccinated animals can be explained on no other ground. These studies seem also to add support to Koch's claim of having solved the problem of having produced a complete immunity in animals by injections of his new tuberculin derived from the crushed body substances of the bacillus, and would lead us to hope that his brilliant results on the subject may soon be confirmed by other experimenters (Trudeau, 1897, p. 1850).

Trudeau's final experiments lasted four years and consumed much of his time, as well as that of Drs. Baldwin, Hewetson, Nelson, and Wilder (Trudeau

1898a, 1899, 1898b). Antitoxins for tetanus and diphtheria had been developed by 1890, and others had claimed to develop immunity in rabbits by injecting serum from immunized dogs. The experiments involved "four sheep, three asses, twelve fowls, eighteen rabbits, and four hundred and fifty guinea-pigs" (1898b, p. 120). These numbers indicate that the new "Saranac Laboratory for the Study of Tuberculosis" was a well-funded facility. The requirements of science had increased in two decades and Trudeau's wealthy friends were supplying that support.

Trudeau described two sets of studies. "The studies included in Part I relate to the methods adopted by us in attempts at producing the sought-for immunity in various animals, and the tests of the germicidal and curative properties which might be possessed by the serum of animals thus immunized. The studies included in Part II relate to tests in animals of the antitoxic power of serums in tuberculin poisoning" (Trudeau, 1897b, p. 114).

Each animal was inoculated with a specific type of bacilli:

- filtrate of tubercle bacillus cultures on thymus bouillon
- tubercle bacillus of increasing virulence
- increasing doses of tuberculin
- living non-virulent cultures of tubercle bacillus
- virulent living cultures of tubercle bacillus
- dead cultures of non-virulent tubercle bacilli on thymus bouillon
- alkaline extracts of the bacilli with dead bacilli (Trudeau, 1897b, p. 115).

From each animal blood serum was taken. The effect of the serum on healthy animals was studied. Tuberculous animals were treated with the serum to see how it affected the course of disease and temperature. And the germicidal influence of the serum was tested in vivo and in vitro. The results were discouraging. "Only one [serum] indicated slight antitoxic power. . . . None of the serums appeared to prevent the local or general reaction from small doses of tuberculin; nor influence the temperature of the tuberculous animals" (Trudeau, 1897b, p. 121). Despite these results, they concluded: "Disappointing as these results may seem, the writers feel that, in the light of recent contributions by Ehrlich, Wasserman, and Behring to our knowledge of the mechanism of immunity and antitoxin production in the body, the outlook for an efficient tuberculosis antitoxin is by no means a hopeless one" (Trudeau, 1897b, p. 121). Trudeau's optimism led him to hope for some method of producing immunity. Baldwin said that between 1892 and 1900 Trudeau conducted or directed "fifty different attempts to immunize animals with dead and living bacilli of varying virulence, and with varying dosage intervals, etc." (Baldwin, 1916, p. 100). From a letter Trudeau wrote in the summer of the year he died, 1915, to the *British Journal of Tuberculosis,* Baldwin quoted, "Nothing has occurred to diminish my faith in the value of tuberculin treatment—a faith which has been

manifested by my continuing its use uninterruptedly in my practice at the
Adirondack Cottage Sanitarium ever since it was discovered, and through all
the long years I stood nearly alone in my medical environment in its advocacy.
If skillfully used, tuberculin stimulates the defensive resources of the organism
and is a valuable adjunct to our treatment in many cases" (Baldwin, 1916, p.
100).

But the search for immunity in humans eluded Edward Trudeau. In the lecture
delivered at Johns Hopkins Hospital on May 1, 1899, he described "the most
promising lines for future work in relation to the etiology, pathology, prophylaxis, bacteriology, diagnosis and treatment of tuberculosis" (Trudeau, 1899a,
p. 121). He still insisted that relative artificial immunity had been produced,
even though the animals eventually died of chronic tuberculosis. Trudeau began
to re-define tuberculosis. "Tuberculosis does not belong to that class of infectious diseases which kill by acute toxemia, but to the class to which syphilis,
actinomycosis, and leprosy also belong, and which destroy life, not only by the
chronic and long-continued systemic poisoning they produce, but by the
pathogenic changes brought about through the localization and growth of the
germs in organs necessary to life" (Trudeau, 1898b, p. 112). The Johns Hopkins
lecture recited a long list of vexing questions confronting the tuberculosis
researcher. It is doubtful that Trudeau was overwhelmed by the list, but he did
not publish specific experimental research from the laboratory again.

For many years Trudeau's laboratory provided a variety of tuberculous
cultures (human, avian, bovine, turtle, frog, rabbit) to the laboratories of
researchers in this country and abroad. From the "Record of Cultures Furnished
to Physicians and Laboratories" from his Saranac Laboratory it is obvious that
Trudeau shared cultures with the leading medical researchers of the day. Most
medical schools did not have laboratories until after the Flexner report of 1911.
A partial list of researchers to whom Trudeau sent cultures of live bacilli,
tuberculin, and so on reveals that he was in communication with the best labs
in North America.

1894, 1989 A. C. Abbott, University of Pennsylvania, Laboratory of Hygiene

1894, 1897, 1900 T. M. Prudden, Columbia, Physicians and Surgeons

1896, 1898, 1904, 1907 H. I. Klopp, Cornell, N.Y. State Veterinary College

1897 C. J. Bartlett, Yale Medical School

1897 W. H. Bergtold, Denver

1897 W. M. L. Coplin, Laboratory of Jefferson Medical College and Hospital

1897 W. S. Halsted, Johns Hopkins Hospital

1904 E. W. Archibald, Royal Victoria Hospital, Montreal

1905 H. S. Custian, Harvard Medical School

1907 V. Bowditch, Boston

1907 L. Buerget, Mt. Sinai Hospital, N.Y.

1907 C. A. Covell, University of Syracuse Medical Department

1908 A. C. Klebs, Chicago

1910 O. T. Avery, Hoagland Laboratory, Brooklyn

1911 C. R. Austrair, Phthysis Dispensary, Johns Hopkins Medical School

1914 H. L. Amoss, Rockefeller Institute, N.Y.

1916 S. A. Harvey, Harvard Medical School

1916 H. I. Klopp, Homeopathic State Hospital, Allentown, Penn.

This illustrates that Trudeau's laboratory was connected to a network of allopathic and homeopathic researchers who presumably shared information. In his correspondence are letters that indicate Trudeau engaged in scholarly exchanges.

The following exchange with von Ruck (whom his friend Alfred Worcester described as "worse than an old rascal" in 1904) indicated that Trudeau could be impatient and not always accommodating. Karl von Ruck had worked with A. C. Klebs and wrote as the Director of Winyah Sanitarium, Asheville, North Carolina. He requested "a sample of the (antiphthisin) which you made . . . [and] a copy of the daily records of your animal experiments and findings in postmortem examination, and will be pleased to pay for the hire of necessary labor to make copies (December 12, 1895, correspondence).

On December 26, Trudeau replied that there was no antiphthisin left and added, "In regard to the injections and autopsies you speak of, we have them all on the books at the laboratory, as well as the organs of the animals in alcohol, but I cannot see that any good purpose could be served by going again over all the details of the experiment, as I think the facts given in the paper are sufficient, the more so as all the animals, whether treated or untreated, died, and all had gross tubercular lesions" (Trudeau to von Ruck, December 26, 1895). Had Trudeau been inclined he might have invited von Ruck to visit the lab, read the books and examine the specimens for himself.

Baldwin took over the direction of the laboratory, and Trudeau turned his efforts to the sanitarium and the movement to prevent tuberculosis.

11

Sanitorium and Outdoor Care

In the late 1800s epidemics of disease like influenza and cholera could surge over a population, causing widespread disease and death. This was especially true in cities with large concentrations of poverty where people were crowded and living in unhygienic conditions. In 1892 the American people experienced a lesson in public health and hygiene. When a cholera epidemic erupted in Hamburg, Germany, several passenger ships carried infected people to New York City. The ships were quarantined and those with cholera isolated and tested by the new bacteriological laboratory of the New York City Board of Health set up by Dr. Hermann Biggs. Because of these efforts, the city was spared an epidemic of cholera and the needless loss of many lives (Harvey, 1986). Trudeau had experienced his own lesson in the effectiveness of quarantine when a flu epidemic hit Saranac Lake (1890a). Now that germs were understood by most citizens, people with tuberculosis were discriminated against because they were contagious. They were refused admission in general hospitals and no alternatives were available. Wealthy families could employ a nurse in their home or escape to some spa, but this was beyond the reach of the majority.

In the lecture at Johns Hopkins Trudeau argued for specially constructed open-air sanitoria as the best chance for recovery. But these should be experimental facilities to study the best methods of treatment (Trudeau, 1899, p. 125). Trudeau argued,

If we recognize that tuberculosis in its earlier stages and more chronic forms is a curable disease, and that in its more acute types or when far advanced, its victims have, on humanitarian grounds, a claim to be cared for; if we also bear in mind that most tuberculosis patients are a danger to the community in which they live, it is evident that, in dealing with tuberculosis in the poorer class of patients, the two main problems to be met are to furnish one class with a place where they can be treated in the earlier stages of their disease with a reasonable prospect of success, and to afford the other class an asylum where they can be properly cared for until they die, and that by so doing the spread of infection in the community will be greatly lessened (Trudeau, 1897d, pp. 276–77).

Arguing that England had established separate hospitals for consumptives, and the death rate from tuberculosis had fallen, Trudeau suggested:

Such hospitals should be located outside but within convenient distances of large cities, and should consist of one or more pavilions connected by galleries, and so constructed that each ward can easily be kept clean and free from dust according to modern methods, while an ample air space is allowed for each patient, and the most thorough ventilation with an abundance of sunlight is secured.

Such institutions would afford the unfortunate victims of the disease a place where they can be cared for when helpless, and where they would no longer be a menace to the health of the community. The large amount of infectious material now scattered by such patients among the closely packed inhabitants of crowded tenements could be easily cared for by this plan and rendered harmless, and it would seem reasonable to hope that such hospitals would decrease the number of cases occurring each year (Trudeau, 1897d, p. 277).

Trudeau publicized his design for a sanitorium consisting of small cottages.

This plan of construction separates the patients as much as possible from one another, and affords each individual so large an air space as to make it difficult, when rigid precautions as to the care of the expectoration are enforced, for the buildings to become contaminated. Besides it affords patients a regular walk to and from their meals, which are served in the main building, encourages them to lead an outdoor life, and allows them to select as companions those who are congenial to them (Trudeau, 1897d, p. 277).

A separate infirmary was necessary.

Should any patient in one of the cottages become rapidly worse or be taken suddenly ill, he is at once removed to the infirmary, where every convenience for his care and proper treatment is at hand. The separation of those who are failing rapidly or are acutely sick from the comparatively well, not only furnishes the former with the constant and necessary attention and nursing which they require, but withdraws them from the daily observation of their more fortunate cottage mates, and prevents in these the depression of spirits which would otherwise occur from the contact with the very sick (Trudeau, 1897d, p. 278).

He argued for rigid measures for the care of expectoration and cited a study by Dr. Irwin H. Hance (1897), one of his resident physicians. That study showed that in only one cottage where a patient had been "careless in the matter of expectoration" was there dust that contained tubercle bacilli. By good hygiene patients and staff could be protected from infection.

Trudeau wanted every sanitorium equipped with a laboratory not only for diagnosis of difficult cases, but for studying the disease. The work of the Sanitarium Laboratory was supported by Mrs. Harriman's contribution of $25,000 in 1911 and Mrs. Russell Sage's contributions of $25,000 in 1911 and 1912 (Annual Report, 1911, 1912). He argued that physicians should make a diagnosis of tuberculosis as early as possible, by microscopic examination of sputum and use of the tuberculin test. Even if the patient appears healthy, he should be "told the grave nature of his malady and an immediate removal from his surroundings should be urged, while it is explained to him that the best and possibly the only chance of restoration lies in prompt action and the adoption of thorough measures" (Trudeau, 1897c, p. 279). He recognized that many patients could not afford to take this advice and go to a sanitorium, but he argued they should be provided for.

It will be justly urged that in a great majority of cases among the poorer classes it is absolutely impossible for the patient to follow the advice given. This is greatly to be regretted; and while it in no way relieves the physician of the responsibility of making an early diagnosis, and advising prompt and radical measures to those who can afford to follow his advice, it is a strong plea for attempting to provide for a greater number of these unfortunates, sanitaria where they can find the climatic and hygienic surroundings necessary for the treatment of their disease as soon as its presence is recognized (Trudeau, 1897d, p. 279).

By 1906, the endowment of the sanitarium had grown to $400,000 (Rockefeller to Harriman, December 6, 1906). Many patients were employed on the grounds by 1912, partly because the public feared such work. The goal of sanitorium care was "to improve the patient's nutrition and increase his resistance to the disease, by placing him under the most favorable environment obtainable. The main elements of such an environment are an invigorating climate, an open-air life, rest, coupled with the careful regulation of the daily habits, and an abundant supply of nutritious food" (Trudeau, 1897d, p. 279).

At the beginning patients should undergo "absolute rest" in the open air for as long as it takes to return their temperature to normal. Only then may they exercise, but never enough to raise the temperature. Trudeau then made an estimate of his results.

The exact results obtained by the combined climatic and sanitarium treatment are difficult to express in figures, because these results are greatly influenced by the class of cases accepted for treatment, and the classification of these cases is purely arbitrary. In addition, the term "cure," as indicating the results obtained, can be used only in a relative sense. If, however, all attempt at classification is abandoned, and the gross results obtained in all the patients admitted to the sanitarium are considered, it may be stated approximately that twenty percent are apparently cured, and that in thirty percent more the disease is more or less permanently arrested. If the most favorable of all the cases admitted are separated under the term "incipient," the proportion of cures obtained would be as high as from thirty to thirty-five per cent, and the importance of making an early diagnosis and of the immediate application of radical measures is strongly emphasized by this experience (Trudeau, 1897d, p. 281).

This talk at the New York Academy of Medicine was the first of many Trudeau gave selling sanitoria as a method of care. By 1897, the Adirondack Cottage Sanitarium was a well equipped, well-run facility. It served as a prototype for the 500 tuberculosis sanitoria that were to be constructed around the country.

The paper described above (Trudeau, 1897d) became the groundwork for four more papers (Trudeau, 1899b, 1900a, 1900b, 1900c). Trudeau updated some sections as new equipment became available. He was especially anxious to motivate apathetic physicians to diagnose tuberculosis as early as possible (Trudeau, 1899b, p. 138).

Trudeau gave clear suggestions for discovering tuberculosis in its incipient stage:

The occurrence of slight haemoptysis as an initial symptom, and before any constitutional impairment is noticeable, should be a most fortunate event for the patient, and in many cases proves to be the first symptom of pulmonary tuberculosis. . . .

The fully developed chest or comparatively robust appearance of many patients with early tuberculosis often proves misleading to the examiner, and induces him to relax his vigilance, to minimize the symptoms, and to wait for further developments. Too great reliance is, perhaps, placed on the physical signs alone, which at first may be either absent or can be detected only by the trained ear, and too little importance is attached to the study of the history and the rational symptoms. In insidious cases lassitude, some loss of appetite, a little quickening of the pulse-rate, a temperature reaching occasionally 99.5 to 100 degrees at irregular intervals, with or without slight loss of weight, are a group of symptoms which usually attracts little attention, but which should be regarded with suspicion. And if, in addition to these, morning pallor, disappearing towards evening, some cough, prolonged expiration, or even impairment of vesicular murmur are noted, the patient should be closely watched, every effort made to obtain more positive evidence; and if it's not obtainable otherwise, the aid of laboratory methods in helping to clear up the diagnosis should not be neglected. If there is expectoration, and the presence of the bacillus cannot be detected by repeated and thorough examinations, a positive conclusion can often be reached within three weeks by inoculation of the expectoration in the guinea-pig. A careful examination with a good X-ray machine and the fluoroscope will often confirm the diagnosis by showing the diaphragm to be higher on the suspected side, or its excursion diminished on one or both sides, and in many cases a slight shadow can also be detected at the site of the suspected lesion. . . .

If additional and more conclusive evidence is required, the tuberculin test should be applied (Trudeau, 1899b, pp. 138–39).

He then described his method of administering the tuberculin test (see p. 143).

The sanitarium had recently purchased an X-ray machine, a new device on the market. Trudeau had traveled to Boston to study with a Dr. Williams and learned to read X-ray pictures (Trudeau, 1900c, p. 47).

What Trudeau and his colleagues meant by the open-air treatment is revealed in the following quotation.

The invigorating influence of a life spent constantly out of doors for many months can hardly be overrated. To remain, in most cases, the greater part of the time quietly sitting, well wrapped up, out of doors in all weathers, is one of the main duties imposed upon every patient at the sanitarium, and, irksome as such a course would at first seem, it is, in a majority of cases, faithfully carried out by them after their timidity and prejudices as to its danger have been gradually overcome by the benefit derived in their own persons.

The outdoor method is applied to all patients, but the details of the treatment, and, above all, the amount of exercise allowed in carrying it out, are regulated by the activity of the patient's disease, his nutritive condition, and more especially his temperature record. Thus, the few infirmary cases who may be suffering from progressive tuberculosis processes or cheesy pneumonias, and running high temperatures, are carried outdoors daily, and kept there in a recumbent position in bed or on a lounge the greater part of the day, while those who have less fever and are improving are allowed to sit up in steamer chairs on the veranda and to walk about the infirmary, but not to go over to their meals in the main building until their temperature record and improved condition warrant it, when they are returned to their cottages. In the class of cases which is represented by the inmates of the cottages the temperature rarely goes above a hundred in the afternoon, or they are entirely apyretic. The former are ordered to remain quiet out of doors during the afternoon, when slight fever is apt to occur, and to walk to their meals in the main building, but not to go off the grounds; while the apyretic cases are generally allowed, so long as they live out of doors and obey rules, to go where they please, and while under daily observation, to take as much exercise as their condition seems to render permissible (Trudeau, 1899b, pp. 140–42).

Visitors who were accustomed to seeing sick people in hospital wards had a hard time accepting these comfortable conditions. Often they asked where the sick people were. Except for the strict emphasis on rest, the sanitarium was very similar to resort life in the Adirondacks, like that Trudeau had experienced at Paul Smith's. He did not agree with some who advocated exercise:

It is much better . . . always to err on the side of over-caution in prescribing active exercise to tuberculous patients, and I feel confident that many lives are constantly sacrificed to a deep-rooted and very general misconception which exists in the lay, and to a great extent in the professional mind as well, in regard to the advantages of active exercise in this disease. If there is any one rule that should be generally applied to the treatment of tuberculosis, it is, that when any degree of fever is present the course of the disease will be injuriously affected in proportion to the amount of active exercise the patient is allowed to take. Still further, I constantly see an apparently quiescent and arrested process fanned into renewed and often uncontrollable activity by one single over-exertion. . . .

Absolute rest, so long as it is taken in the open air, is the best measure at our command to reduce the pyrexia of tuberculosis and to conserve the patient's energies, and should be persisted in for some time after the afternoon fever has ceased to be present, moderate exercise again being allowed only with caution (Trudeau, 1899b, p. 142).

Trudeau relied on rest, fresh air, and nutrition as the primary factors in treatment. Drugs were used sparingly, and then only to relieve symptoms, much as Alonzo Clark had taught thirty years earlier.

Alcoholics are never prescribed in early cases as a part of the treatment. Little stress is laid on the administration of drugs except when necessary to relieve symptoms, but cod-liver oil, the hypophosphites, and arsenic are very gradually made use of. Creosote is prescribed in small doses only, and in cases where cough and profuse expectoration seem to indicate its administration, or where its tentative use has shown that it improves rather than impairs the patient's appetite and digestion (Trudeau, 1899b, p. 143).

Trudeau described his use of Koch's tuberculin. After the formula became available, he made his own tuberculin at the Saranac Laboratory. There is some indication that Trudeau did not trust the quality of tuberculin supplied by Koch. When Koch produced a new TR tuberculin, Trudeau and Baldwin decided to check it out themselves, with these results: "Although the directions accompanying the bottles of the new TR tuberculin state that it contains ten milligrams of solid substance, if the water and glycerin be evaporated only about four milligrams of solid substance remain" (Trudeau, 1899b, p. 143). Also, they discovered it contained "living tubercle bacilli" and therefore refused to use it.

Finally, Trudeau presented results from the 1897 and 1898 annual reports (see Table 11.1).

For the first time, Trudeau defined his terms:

1. Incipient—Cases in which both the physical and rational signs point to but slight local and constitutional involvement.

2. Advanced—Cases in which the localized disease process is either extensive or in an advanced stage, or where, with a comparatively slight amount of pulmonary involvement, the rational signs point to grave constitutional impairment or to some complication.

3. Far Advanced—Cases in which both the rational and physical signs warrant the term.

4. Apparently Cured—Cases in which the rational signs of phthisis and the bacilli in the expectoration have been absent for at least three months, or who have no expectoration at all, any abnormal physical signs remaining being interpreted as indicative of a healed lesion.

Table 11.1
203 Patients Who Remained an Average of 9 Months

Condition of Patients when admitted		Apparently Cured	Disease Arrested	Improved	Unimproved or Failed	Died
75	Incipient	55	16	2	2	0
84	Advanced	15	38	19	11	1
44	Far Advanced	0	7	19	13	5
203	Total	70	61	40	26	6

> 5. Arrested—Cases in which cough, expectoration, and bacilli are still present, but in which all constitutional disturbance has disappeared for several months, the physical signs being interpreted as indicative of a retrogressive or arrested process (Trudeau, 1899b, pp. 145–60).

Defining these categories was very important if the results of various forms of treatment were to be compared not only at the Adirondack Cottage Sanitarium, but from one sanitorium to another.

Trudeau stressed that these statistics affirmed the importance of making an early diagnosis. "Of the forty-four patients classified as far advanced not a single one recovered, while of the seventy-five who represent the earliest stage at which the disease can be detected, fifty-five, or 73.5 percent, were apparently cured" (Trudeau, 1899b, p. 146).

Trudeau repeated this sanitorium paper several times with minimal changes. In the paper published in the *Medical News* he revised his statistics down a bit, claiming "that 68 percent of the truly incipient cases were discharged as apparently cured, while only 11 percent of the advanced and none of the far advanced cases recovered" (Trudeau, 1900b, p. 852). To further emphasize the importance of early diagnosis he described the following case:

One case which I saw during the earlier part of last summer illustrates these points. Repeated physical examinations by experts of undoubted skill had been negative; the X-ray picture was inconclusive; there was no cough or expectoration, the only symptoms present being some loss of weight and strength, and a temperature which occasionally touched 99.5 degrees F. in the evening. The patient was a physician and insisted on a diagnosis, therefore I advised the tuberculin test. Two milligrams gave a typical reaction. He obtained a year's leave of absence and went West. A few months later he wrote me he had gained twenty pounds, and that no one believed he had ever had tuberculosis. Recently I received a letter from him stating that one morning, after some unusual physical exertion the previous day, he had spit a teaspoonful of blood, and that on being examined by a physician he had been told that there was a slight pleuritic friction-sound behind the right scapula (Trudeau, 1900b, p. 853).

The earlier version of the sanitorium paper had described Trudeau's use of tuberculin as a treatment and given results, but without any control group. In this version data were presented for those treated with tuberculin since 1891 and compared to a control group of patients who received the general treatment and were discharged apparently cured at the same periods of time (see Table 11.2). These figures show a slight trend favoring the tuberculin cases, but are not sufficiently different to be in any way conclusive. Trudeau did not interpret these results as confirming the value of tuberculin treatment. Again, he presented results for 1897–99 (see Table 11.3). These results were essentially the same as had been produced using the 1897–99 data. To answer critics of the sanitorium method, Trudeau added some new data collected by Dr. Baldwin (1900) to these yearly summaries.

I am quite aware that cure in tuberculosis is but a relative term and that time is the only test of cure; a test which becomes more and more discouraging as the period of its application lengthens and we become more familiar with the relapsing nature of the disease. Nevertheless, we have attempted to determine as far as was practicable the permanency of the results obtained extending over a period of fifteen years to date. Of the 1176 patients discharged alive about one-half are still living, and one-half of this number have been heard from as being perfectly well. This proportion of one-quarter of the whole number covers the entire fifteen years, and the percentage, of course, improves every year as more early cases are admitted. The permanency of the

Table 11.2
Tuberculin Treatment Compared to Controls Receiving the General Treatment

	Tuberculin Treated	General Treatment
Not traced	3	3
Well; returned to work in former surroundings	29	21
Well; living out-of-door life in other good climates	7	10
Well; not working	5	5
Relapsed (living)	1	6
Relapsed (dead)	4	5
Died insane	1	0
Total	50	50

Table 11.3
Patients Who Remained an Average of 8.75 Months

Condition of Patients When Admitted		Apparently Cured	Disease Arrested	Improved	Unimproved or Failed	Died
Incipient	113	82[1]	25	4	2	0
Advanced	151	27[2]	67	43	13	1
Far Advanced	59	0	12	26	16	5
Total	323	109[3]	104	73	31	6

[1]72.566%   [2]17.880%   [3]33.746%

recoveries depends necessarily a good deal on the environment to which the patient returns. If he is obliged to go back to a laborious life or an indoor occupation he is much more likely to relapse than if it is possible for him to return to a good climate and an outdoor existence (Trudeau, 1900b, p. 857).

Trudeau was expressing his own life story. Whenever he was overworked he became feverish and his cough returned, especially after 1900. He was making a political argument, as well. "The attempt to cure pulmonary tuberculosis by institutional treatment and the practical demonstration which it has given of the possibility of accomplishing this in many cases have cast a ray of light on one of the darkest problems which confront medical science and have proved an object-lesson which has, perhaps, not been without influence in creating the present popular demand that the State supplement private philanthropy in the establishment of similar institutions under its control" (Trudeau, 1900b, p. 857). He provided evidence for and advocated the construction of sanitoria throughout the country as one of the factors in the crusade against the great white plague, tuberculosis.

The sanitorium article was repeated in the *Zeitschrift fur Tuberkulose unde Heilstattenwesen* (vol. 1, 1900a), a German journal for tuberculosis and sanitorium design. Aware of political realities, he titled it "The First People's Sanitarium in America for the Treatment of Pulmonary Tuberculosis." The paper was presented again in May 1990 at the Association of American Physicians Meeting. In this version, Trudeau cited more evidence that rest was essential. "Murphy's proposed treatment, which consists in putting the diseased lung completely at rest by introducing nitrogen gas into the pleural cavity, is another proof by the surgeon of the value of absolute rest" (Trudeau, 1900c, p. 39). In the discussion that followed, Trudeau admitted that he had not yet tried Dr. Murphy's suggestion. He did experience pneumothorax in April 1912 and claimed he was helped (1900c, p. 47).

Parts of the sanitorium paper were used in other papers. He stressed "The Importance of a Recognition of the Significance of Early Tuberculosis in Relation to Treatment" (Trudeau 1901b, 1901c). This was essential if tuberculosis were to be controlled. He gave this paper to the Association of American Physicians in May 1901, and it was published in the *Medical News* in June. To his colleagues at the association he added a few things to the original discussion of his methods of diagnosis (pp. 106–107). He was especially concerned that local doctors did not recognize the early signs of tuberculosis and were unwilling to disrupt patient's lives.

In spite of every effort, much difficulty is experienced in securing incipient cases for admission to the Adirondack Cottage Sanitarium, and 70 percent of applicants give histories which make it evident that some of the symptoms of tuberculosis have been present for from one to three years before they were advised to apply for admission. The examiners for the Massachusetts State Hospital for the Treatment of Tuberculosis refuse about 60 percent of all who apply because their disease is too far advanced. About the same proportion is refused in our examinations at Saranac Lake, and of the remaining 40 percent admitted not more than one-half are really incipient cases (Trudeau, 1901d, p. 116).

Trudeau contrasted this American experience with evidence from Germany. "Dr. Wicher, at the Berlin Congress, stated that at his sanatorium near Goebersdorf, of the cases which he classes as 'initial state,' and which were discharged as cured in 1896–1897–1898, 97 percent were still at work on January 1, 1899, while on the same date, of those who when they entered the sanatorium were classed as 'advanced phthisis with destructive process,' and discharged during the same years, 77 percent were dead" (Trudeau, 1901c, p. 117). Dr. Baldwin's statistics (1900) could not be compared with these, but Trudeau envied such results and expected they could be achieved if he could convince physicians to identify early tuberculosis.

Another section of the sanitorium article spawned two papers on the general topic of "artificial immunity" (Trudeau, 1903, 1904). At the eighteenth annual meeting of the Association of American Physicians, Trudeau read "Artificial Immunity in Experimental Tuberculosis" (Trudeau, 1903a, 1903b). This paper is a combination of work that he had published earlier (Trudeau 1890c, 1893, 1894, 1897b, 1899a; Trudeau and Baldwin, 1895, 1898b, 1899). Having labored in this area for nearly fifteen years, Trudeau was well qualified to write the history of attempts to demonstrate artificial immunity in laboratory animals. He described recent work by Baldwin with calves and his own work using another attenuated tubercle bacillus. With guinea pigs, he demonstrated "relative immunity," the control dying in an average of fifty-five days, while some experimental animals lived "over a year" (Trudeau, 1903a, p. 105). Trudeau displayed jars of rabbit lungs inoculated with "attenuated R.1 tubercle bacillus culture" and killed at various stages. Recognizing his own subjectivity, he had Dr. Hodenpyl analyze the lungs. He concluded: "It is evident . . . that the violent reaction of the tissues to the virulent inoculation in protected animals tends to end in an aborting of the progressive tuberculous process, in the partial absorption of the morbid products, in destruction of the bacilli, and a more or less complete return to normal as far as this is possible" (Trudeau, 1903a, p. 107). Trudeau hoped that the results would produce more studies that minimize the "violent reaction" and produce "a more durable immunization." But at this point the dangers of the immunizing process were still too great to warrant tests on humans.

From the sanitorium paper Trudeau started another paper summarizing "Studies on the Tuberculin Reaction" conducted between 1900 and 1904. This paper was interrupted by another tragedy.

TRAGEDY AGAIN

The Trudeaus' son, Ned, had led a happy and successful life. After four years at St. Paul's School and four more at Yale, he went to the College of Physicians and Surgeons, graduating in 1900. Following service as an intern at Presbyterian Hospital in New York, Ned returned to Saranac Lake to work with his father.

He intended to settle here and help me with my work, but I did all I could to dissuade him from this. With his wonderful charm, his very thorough education, and his vigorous health, I saw a much more brilliant future for him elsewhere. I was beginning already to realize the stigma with which the world stamps everything and everybody connected with tuberculosis, and I saw no reason why Ned should voluntarily assume this burden. I was therefore overjoyed when my good friend Dr. Walter B. James offered him a place in his office in New York City, with every opportunity there for advancement in his profession, and it seemed to me and to all my friends that a very bright future was before him (Trudeau, 1915, pp. 272–73).

We can only guess that Edward wanted his son to have the prominent career in New York City which tuberculosis had forced him to relinquish. Dr. James had been a good friend for many years and served on the board of the sanitarium. Shortly after Ned married Hazel Martyn, "a talented artist and a very beautiful woman, the young married couple settled in New York, and Ned was soon launched into practice and other medical activities through his connection with Dr. James" (Trudeau, 1915, p. 275). In the spring of 1904 the Trudeaus received a telegram from Dr. James telling them Ned had suddenly been overcome by an acute pneumonia and urging them to come by the evening train. After five days the crisis had passed and Dr. Janeway said he would recover and in ten days they could take him back to Saranac Lake to recuperate. But that afternoon "he died suddenly of a heart clot." Trudeau's description of the support of friends and the community illustrated their esteem not only for Ned, but for the family and the "beloved physician" as well.

Through all these terrible, dark days, however, the tender sympathy and love of our friends and his friends shone, and shines even now like a soft light in the midst of impenetrable gloom. Everyone who new Ned and knew us tried to show their love for him, and that touched us and helped us bear our own suffering. . . .

Among many others, Dr. James, Dr. Linsly Williams, Mr. Harriman and Lawrence Aspinwall were with us through all that terrible evening when Ned lay dead in the next room, and they did everything that love and sympathy and helpful friendship could do to steady us and relieve us in doing what had to be done.

The next afternoon at the Grand Central Station we found two cars Mr. Harriman had arranged for, attached to the Adirondack Train. In one Ned's body lay, buried under a roomful of flowers and surrounded by his Yale chums, who sat up all night by him as the car sped through the darkness toward the mountains and the little churchyard under the tall pines at Paul Smith's. The other car was prepared for us and many friends.

The next morning broke clear and beautiful, and as we approached the church it was evident the whole country had come to show their love for the young man who had lived his boyhood and most of his life among them. Streams of carriages came from Saranac Lake and the surrounding country, and when we reached the churchyard, as at Chatte's funeral, we found Paul Smith and his sons and other faithful friends had covered all the ground from the Church to the grave with flowers and green boughs. The Smiths had thrown open their hotel and provided liberal entertainment all that day for the crowd of people who came. Had Ned been their own son and brother they could not have done more.

But I was to have further proof of the love and esteem in which he was held. A few days later I started out to collect and settle all the bills for the funeral. Everywhere the answer was the same. There was no bill. What they had done, they had done to show their affection for him. This was repeated everywhere, from Paul Smith and his sons, who arranged for the funeral, opened the hotel and provided for a crowd of guests at St. Regis, to the livery-stable men and even the poor hackmen in Saranac Lake, who refused to take money for what they had done—not for money, but to show their affection for him (Trudeau, 1915, pp. 276–77).

It was characteristic of Edward Trudeau to deny that these expressions of love, affection, and esteem were directed to the whole family. And it is doubtful that they would have been so impressive had Dr. and Mrs. Trudeau not expressed similar love for their friends, patients, and neighbors. Trudeau's health had been failing, and Ned's death did not help.

THE TUBERCULIN REACTION

The paper "Studies on the Tuberculin Reaction" was jointly authored with Drs. E. R. Baldwin and H. M. Kinghorn. The goal of these studies was to better understand the "nature and specificity of the tuberculin reaction" that Trudeau had described in the sanitorium paper (see 1899b, p. 139). On corneal tuberculosis in rabbits they demonstrated that the use of tuberculin injections did not produce a spread of the disease (Trudeau, Baldwin, and Kinghorn, 1904, p. 172). When "abscesses produced by subcutaneous injection of living and dead tubercle bacilli were excised," surgically, one rabbit did not show the typical reaction to tuberculin (Trudeau, Baldwin, and Kinghorn, 1904, p. 174). After rabbits with implanted inert capsules of live bacilli did not react to tuberculin, they concluded that "the presence of tubercle bacilli or their substance in the tissues appears necessary to a true tuberculin reaction" (Trudeau, Baldwin, and Kinghorn, 1904, p. 179). Finally, they determined that a consistent tuberculin reaction did not appear in guinea pigs until ten to fifteen days after injection (Trudeau, Baldwin, and Kinghorn, 1904, p. 187).

While his colleagues continued to produce scientific papers at the Saranac Laboratory (seventy papers from 1887 to 1908), Dr. Trudeau had finished his laboratory career. He had produced artificial immunity but nothing that was permanent in animals. Though he used tuberculin in treating patients and thought that it was helpful, it never became a standard procedure. The tuberculin test was widely used for diagnostic purposes. The general method of treating patients by rest, an outdoor life, and good nutrition was adopted throughout the country. Trudeau's research added to his credibility and he became a vocal advocate for education and prevention in the fight against tuberculosis.

PREVENTION

The Henry Phipps Institute during the fall and winter (1903–1904) sponsored lectures to formally inaugurate the "crusade against tuberculosis." Edward Trudeau gave the first lecture, "The History of the Tuberculosis Work at Saranac Lake" (1903c). After describing his use of Brehmer's idea of rest, outdoor living and good nutrition, Trudeau said: "It is interesting to note that this great advance in the treatment of pulmonary tuberculosis took place before Koch's epoch-making discovery of the tubercle bacillus, and has been in no-way influenced and modified by it" (Trudeau, 1903c, p. 770). Though he had spent endless hours in his laboratory trying to kill the bacillus, studying tuberculin, and trying to produce artificial immunity, his general treatment of patients at the sanitarium had essentially been the same from the beginning.

Trudeau recognized that research had scientific as well as publicity and political value. As if to emphasize this he presented the results of treating 165 cases in 1902. "We find that 30 percent were discharged as apparently cured, in 41 percent the disease was arrested, 19 percent the diagnosis was doubtful, and 1 percent died in the institution" (Trudeau, 1903c, p. 773). In addition, to look at the problem of relapse, he described Dr. Lawrason Brown's study of 1,500 cases who had been discharged from two to seventeen years.

434 could not be traced, leaving 1066 which have been traced. Of these 46.7 per cent are living. Of these 31 per cent are known to be well at present, in 6.5 per cent the disease is still arrested, 4 per cent have relapsed, 5.2 per cent are chronic invalids, and 53.3 per cent are dead. As to the influence of the stage of the disease on the permanency of the results obtained, he found 66 per cent of the 258 incipient cases discharged are well at present. Of the 563 advanced cases 28.6 per cent are well, and of the far advanced cases 2.5 per cent only, remain well. . . .

These figures, discouraging as they may seem to those of you who are not familiar with this fatal malady [note his choice of words], emphasize the importance of making an early diagnosis, and teach us exactly to what extent we may count on saving and prolonging life by this method of treatment (Trudeau, 1903c, p. 774).

Again these figures supported Trudeau's sanitorium methods and his continued emphasis upon early diagnosis. As an alternative to certain death, a cure rate of 31 percent was attractive.

Regarding his use of tuberculin as a specific, Trudeau noted that it should be used only in incipient cases and revealed another study by Dr. Brown of cases discharged from 1890 to 1901. "Of the incipient cases which received no tuberculin 61 percent are alive up to date, while of the tuberculin treated incipient cases, 76.7 percent are living today. Thus, it would seem that there is still an appreciable though not very pronounced percentage in favor of the tuberculin treated cases" (Trudeau, 1903c, p. 774).

He described his work at the laboratory and his continued hope for developing "artificial immunity." The changes that the sanitarium had caused in the town of Saranac Lake are described. Trudeau was mayor in 1900–1901.

The village of Saranac Lake has been constantly called upon to adapt itself to new conditions, which have transformed it from a guides' settlement to a busy town and much frequented health resort. For twenty years an ever increasing number of invalids has been steadily settling down in Saranac Lake, and the town has now practically developed into a cottage sanitarium on a large scale in order to meet the requirements of an ever-growing invalid population, belonging to all classes of society, from the affluent to the penniless consumptive (Trudeau, 1903c, p. 778).

The town's Board of Health licensed these cure cottages and encouraged hygienic and preventive practices. A Reception Cottage where consumptives were examined by volunteer community physicians and assisted in finding appropriate lodgings was constructed in 1901. Mentioning the works of "Flick in Philadelphia and Biggs in New York City," he stressed "the more practical methods of prevention which already have lowered the death rate from tuberculosis in New York City, and promise in the future, as they are further developed and more generally adopted, even more brilliant results" (Trudeau, 1903c, p. 779). Ever sensitive to a source of support, Trudeau concluded:

Within the year comes the announcement that a large-hearted man has donated to science and philanthropy a princely sum from the fortune he has acquired in a successful life of business activity, and aided by men of science, has founded the Henry Phipps Institute for the Prevention, Treatment and Study of Tuberculosis, under whose auspices we are gathered here tonight. No one, I am sure, can wish this great work Godspeed more earnestly than I do, or appreciate more thoroughly the glorious future that opens before it in the advancement of knowledge and the relief of human suffering (Trudeau, 1903c, p. 780).

That he was invited to give this paper, to be followed by Osler and Biggs, was recognition that Edward Trudeau was one of the clinical and scientific leaders in tuberculosis.

Further recognition of that fact came in 1904, when he was elected president of the Association of American Physicians and first president of the National Association for the Study and Prevention of Tuberculosis. In the former his clinical and scientific skills were most important, for the latter, his reputation and his political skills were essential. To the Association of American Physicians, Trudeau said little more than that he wanted it to keep its tradition of avoiding AMA pettiness. "Its sessions have ever been free from medical politics and ethical disputes, and the time and talents of its members have been solely devoted to the presentation of original observations and researches, and to the discussions and consideration of scientific medicine in its broadest sense" (Trudeau, 1905c, p. 1).

He wanted the association to continue as a forum where "the clinician and the laboratory worker, the general practitioner and the scientist, might meet on common ground" (Trudeau, 1905c, p. 1).

On March 28, 1904, at the Phipps Institute, about one hundred physicians and laymen were convened by Dr. Lawrence Flick, a Philadelphia physician who had recovered from tuberculosis. They formed a "United States Society for the Study and Prevention of Tuberculosis" (Teller, 1988, pp. 29–30; Bates, 1992). "Trudeau, Biggs, Flick, Welch, Sternberg, Osler and H. B. Jacobs became a committee to develop a constitution and by-laws for the organization. This was accomplished at Biggs home in New York City on June 6, 1904 and the name was changed to the National Association . . . to differentiate it from several previous groups that had been extant since 1892" (Teller, 1988, pp. 27–28). These leaders were the most influential tuberculosis authorities in the country and in electing Edward Trudeau their first president they honored a person who expressed their values.

The address to the National Association for the Study and Prevention of Tuberculosis was necessarily political. The knowledge that had been developed over the years had created the responsibility to act against the great white plague. Study of the disease "had inspired men with new hope and led them to the conviction that since tuberculosis is a communicable disease and its etiological factor has been discovered, it is also to a great extent a preventable one" (Trudeau, 1905a, p. 1). This was the knowledge upon which the organization was based. Its goal was "reduction of the death rate from tuberculosis over all the United States of America." It was patterned after an international association to which most European countries already belonged. Trudeau stressed the "first and greatest need" was education, and when the states were educated they would make the following requirements: "A higher standard of public hygiene and improved conditions of life for the masses; sanitary laws embodying the municipal control of tuberculosis as it is now understood; the segregation of the tuberculous in public institutions and prisons; the establishment of sanatoriums for incipient cases; hospitals for advanced and hopeless ones who cannot be cared for safely at their homes; specially organized dispensaries, laboratories for research, etc." (Trudeau, 1905a, p. 2).

Education about tuberculosis should occur in the public schools, among the masses, and among professionals to

crush the vampire of quackery which preys ever on the misfortunes and ignorance of the poor consumptive, appealing with devilish ingenuity, through specious advertisements of mysterious specifics and sure cures, to his credulity and hope, masquerading under the guise of science and even of philanthropy, in order to wring from him his small savings, and then casting him off, when these have been exhausted and his disease is well advanced, doomed to a lingering death, helpless, hopeless, and a heavy burden on the overtaxed resources of a charitable community (Trudeau, 1905a, p. 2).

Trudeau wanted medical schools to give "special didactic and clinical instruction in advanced methods of making an early diagnosis" so all practitioners could identify "the disease in its incipiency" before the "classical symptoms of pulmonary consumption develop." He suggested the tuberculin test was a valuable tool for this purpose. Next Trudeau emphasized the importance of more research in the United States. He concluded:

On the spirit of a work like this depends its life and success. The motive which has brought you together, and the spirit which has made possible the existence of the National Association, is to my mind the best guarantee of its success; for its work represents the highest type of unselfish human endeavor and the highest aim of a noble profession; mainly the struggle for the existence of others. . . .

If the National Association succeeds in coordinating and binding together in one sustained and well-directed effort, the scattered energies which have sprung into life all over the country, if it can secure the cooperation of the sociologist, the legislator and the philanthropist, if its organization is complete and its members have become imbued with the greater meaning and true spirit of cooperation—a cooperation ever ready to sacrifice selfish aims to the success of a great cause—a cooperation which to the athlete means teamwork and to the soldier discipline—it cannot but prove a powerful instrument in the struggle against tuberculosis in this country.

It has been said—"the degree of civilization of a people will in time be indicated by the figures of its death-rate." If this be so the National Association has indeed a great responsibility; one which it nevertheless seems well fitted to assume (Trudeau, 1905a, p. 3).

In this call to arms Trudeau's values are transparent. His emphasis on unselfishness, helping others, cooperation, and concern for groups of people all reflect themes important in his own life. The National Association became a powerful force in decreasing the tuberculosis mortality rate through hygienic and preventive methods. Eventually research produced a cure, but not in Trudeau's lifetime.

12

The Evolution of Sanitorium Care

From the time the Hunt sisters arrived in the fall of 1884, Trudeau kept case histories on each patient treated at the sanitarium. Usually included was a history of the disease, the patient's occupation and working conditions, and a family history noting any deaths from phthisis. The physical exam revealed the use of all the tools available to the technologically sophisticated physician of the 1880s. The chest (front and back) was examined by stethoscope, and sounds such as rales (abnormal respiratory sounds) were carefully described and located. Pectoriloquy (transmission of the sound of spoken words, indicating excavation of the lung) was often noted. Morning and evening temperatures were sometimes recorded. After Trudeau learned to identify the bacillus, the sputum was examined by microscope. Percussion and palpation were used as well. An eye examination would look for ulcers of the cornea. Finally weight loss and gain during treatment were noted and watched carefully.

As all patients were required to rest and ate the same food in a common dining room as soon as they were allowed out of bed, this important part of the treatment was rarely recorded. Extra milk was recommended between meals for particularly underweight patients, often in connection with a laxative. Cod-liver oil was prescribed for many [as it was presumed to improve body weight]. Patients with high fevers were given quinine, a drug commonly used to reduce the temperature in cases of malaria. For many patients Trudeau would write "commenced inhalations in cabinet" (Figure 12.1). Patients were placed into a cabinet, similar to a telephone booth and asked to inhale a variety of substances introduced as fine sprays or gases. In some cases a 2 to 3 percent

Figure 12.1
Case # 16 Record

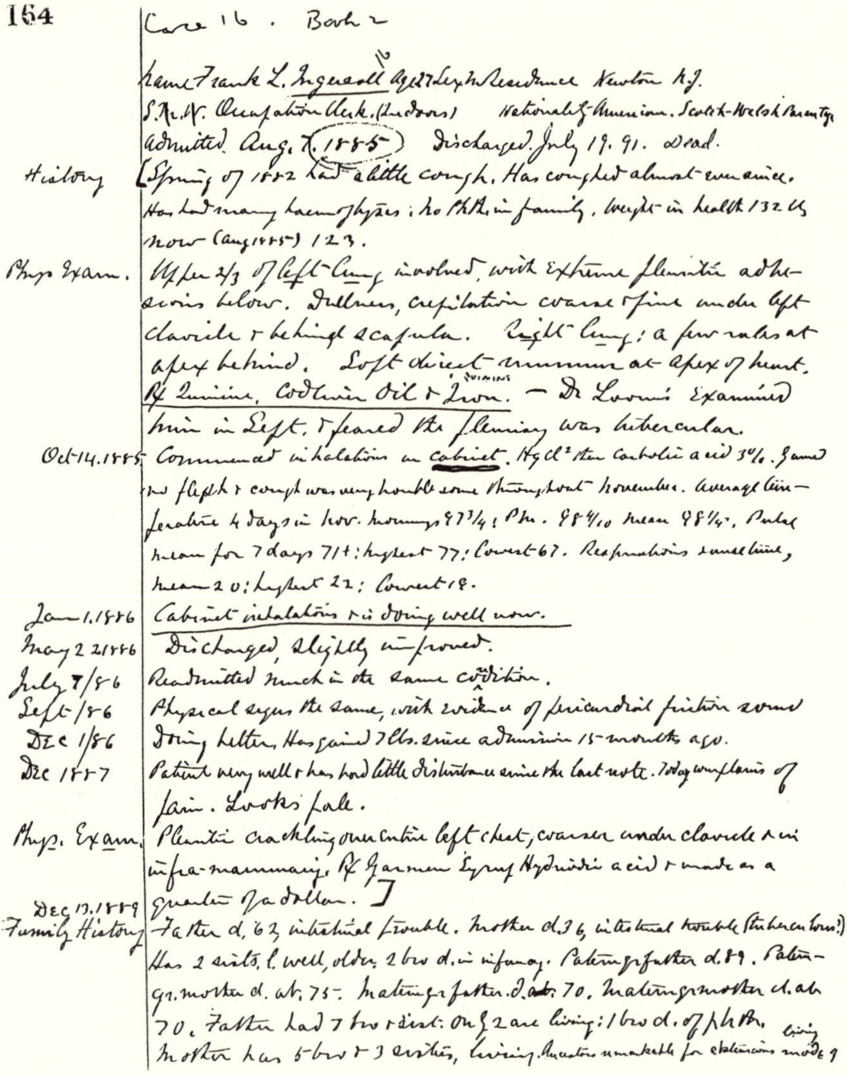

164

Case 16 . Book 2

Name Frank L. Ingersoll Age 27 Residence Newton N.J.
S.R.W. Occupation Clerk (Indoors) Nationality American. Scotch-Welsh Ancestry
Admitted Aug. 7 (1885) Discharged July 19. 91. Dead.

History [Spring of 1882 had a little cough. Has coughed almost ever since.
Has had many haemoptyses; no Phthisis in family. Weight in health 132 lbs
now (aug 1885) 123.

Phys. Exam. Upper 2/3 of left lung involved, with extreme pleuritic adhesions below. Dullness, crepitation coarse & fine under left clavicle & behind scapula. Right lung: a few rales at apex behind. Soft direct murmur at apex of heart. Of Quinine, Codliver Oil & Iron. — Dr Loomis examined him in Sept, & feared the pleurisy was tubercular.

Oct.14.1885 Commenced inhalation in cabinet. Hy Cl & then Carbolic acid 3%. Gained in flesh & cough was very troublesome throughout November. Average temperature 4 days in Nov. mornings 97¼; P.M. 98 4/10 mean 98¼. Pulse mean for 7 days 71½: highest 77: lowest 67. Respirations same time, mean 20; highest 22: lowest 18.

Jan 1.1886 Cabinet inhalations &c doing well now.

May 2 2 1886 Discharged, slightly improved.

July 7/86 Readmitted much in the same condition.

Sept/86 Physical signs the same, with evidence of pericardial friction sound.

Dec 1/86 Doing better, Has gained 7 lbs since admission 15 months ago.

Dec 1887 Patient very well & has had little disturbance since the last note. Today complains of pain. Looks pale.

Phys. Exam. Pleuritic crackling over entire left chest, coarser under clavicle & infra-mammary. Of Garmen Syrup Hydriodic acid & made as a quarter of a dollar.

Dec 13.1889
Family History Father d. 63, intestinal trouble. Mother d. 36, intestinal trouble (tubercular?) Has 2 sisters, l. well, older; 2 bros d. in infancy. Paternal grandfather d. 89. Paternal grandmother d. at 75. Maternal grandfather d. at 70. Maternal grandmother d. ab 70. Father had 7 bros & sisters. Only 2 are living; 1 bro d. of phth. Mother has 5 bros & 3 sisters, living. Ancestors remarkable for robustness mode?

solution of carbolic acid was inhaled for two to eight minutes a day. Creosote or wood smoke distillate, an antiseptic, was inhaled also.

A patient who was treated at the sanitarium in 1886 wrote her impressions in 1919. She described the physical facilities as well as some of the treatments.

We landed February 17th, during the worst blizzard the Adirondacks had experienced in 23 years, the natives said. The buffalo coats (which were general property of the Sanitarium and worn by everybody) did not appear with the stage (a covered sleigh) that met us at Loon Lake, consequently we nearly perished, and the rough ride made one of our party of four desperately sick. . . .

Our arrival at the Main building, the center of the institution, revealed a big open fire, and supper being just over, the 15, or less, patients were gathered round it. Later on we were shown to our cottage, "the little Red." A fire burned in the soap stone stove and the lamp was lighted, but no one slept that wild night for the fury of the storm. . . .

The Sanitarium consisted of three cottages for women and (I think) two for men and the Main building. The outhouse was up on the hill above the back of the Main building a little, approached by a walk of rough stone slabs. The position of it seems a little contrary to modern theories, but as there was no well near it perhaps it was all right.

The Sanitarium had no water supply—only what was carried by hand from a pump. The toilet was as said, outdoors, and a new sand flow had lately been installed. You pulled something and sand ran down is my recollection of it [Indoor toilets were installed in 1891]. . . .

We had plenty to eat, milk and eggs galore, furnished by cows and chickens on the place. One Scotch girl used to drink eleven glasses of milk a day, her name was Neal or Mac Neal.

We had in the front hall a huge boxlike affair known as "the cabinet." It had glass partitions. The patients sat inside and inhaled certain medicated gases or artificial oxygen of some sort as part of the cure. Mr. Ingersoll administered it. [Frank L. Ingersoll, age 27, was admitted August 7, 1885, discharged on May 2, 1886, and readmitted July 7, 1886. He assisted Trudeau for several years until his death on July 19, 1891 (case # 16, Book 2, page 164)].

Trudeau wrote this about Ingersoll:

I had another and unexpected helper at this time Mr. Frank Ingersoll, a medical student. [His occupation is listed in the case book as Clerk (indoors)] Though very ill, he at once took in the situation and filled a big place at the Sanitarium. The patients looked upon him as a doctor, and no one could have taken a more devoted or unselfish interest in everything connected with the institution. He taught me the first great lesson I learned in the conquest of Fate by acquiescence. Alone in the world, among strangers, poor, stricken with what he knew to be a fatal disease, in constant physical weakness and suffering, he never complained and forgot himself in helping others. Always cheerful, always helpful, he worked uncomplainingly until his sudden death from hemorrhage. His example taught me a great lesson, and was a great stimulus to me at this discouraging time. If he was not discouraged, why should I be? (Trudeau, 1915, p. 195).

The letter continued,

Flower beds around the Main building and a row of Nasturtiums beneath the big porch made an attractive appearance but I can yet hear and see patients thoughtlessly expectorate over the rail. Only the very ill used sputum cups (of blue glass). I never needed a cup, but I can see those others yet. Patients were mostly protegés of wealthy people who paid the $15.00 a week necessary, and it was decidedly a mixed society that of necessity formed an intimate family. Teachers, housemaids, farm hands, sporting men and young ladies like Amie and myself, and two other sisters whose name was Long I think.

There was a treatment an employment of sulphuratted hydrogen gas (used experimentally I am sure) by a patient known as Mrs. Lynch. She and her husband were plain Irish people and she left little children home somewhere. This treatment permeated the entire settlement with an odor decidedly akin to very rotten eggs.

We walked over the hill down to the village, and it frequently took half the Sanitarium population to go and purchase a spool of thread, illustrating how time hung on our hands. In winter we rode anywhere that someone had started a road. In spring we found ourselves going over fence tops and the lakes appearing where we had ridden. The daily ride, one party in the mornings and another in the afternoons, wearing the same [buffalo] coats and with hot bricks at our feet made a pleasant diversion.

Of mosquitos I might write a chapter. We had netting all over our beds but that was all. We undressed after crawling under the net carefully. We hung tar or pennyroyal or kerosene cloths on the head board, but between the odors and the incessant singing of the horde "varmints" on the outside, sleep was oftimes long in coming. Black flies were not so serious as they seldom came inside.

In winter we often waded into the forest, thigh deep in snow to cut birch bark and to pierce the spruce gum blisters, spruce gum being said to be a "cure." The maple sugar season furnished much entertainment. In summer, the arrival of the picturesque stage with its four horses and its mail was the real event of the day.

We did not see a great deal of Dr. Trudeau, he came about twice a week! There was an assistant physician whose name I have forgotten. Toward the end of the year I was sent down to the Smith farm house on the road and boarded there for two months (Carolyn Pentland Lindsay, case # 54, March 8, 1919, letter to Dr. Heise at Trudeau Sanitarium).

As this letter indicated, the sanitarium was quite a relaxed place, a middle-class version of Paul Smith's resort, costing only $5 a week at the beginning. Trudeau was struggling to build the sanitarium and had problems with an adequate supply of drinking water and a drainage ditch that created unpleasant odors. These practical difficulties seemed to discourage him in the beginning. He wrote,

I had no definite idea just what to do and very little money with which to do anything. I could not afford a doctor at the institution, and had to do the medical work myself, driving in summer fourteen miles from Paul Smith's and fourteen miles back at each visit. I had no nurse nor anyone to direct the patients and encourage them. When they were taken acutely ill with complications I had no infirmary to send them to, and no one to carry their meals and nurse them in their cottages. I used to hire lumbermen and guides to care for the bed-ridden men patients and any old woman I could get to look after the women, and these were very expensive and not very efficient help. In cases of severe hemorrhage these improvised nurses would become panic-stricken and escape from the sick-room, and often no amount of eloquence on my part would induce them to return. On the rare occasions when anybody died I had to come over and take charge of the situation in person, as the entire establishment was thrown into such a panic that I feared they would all desert in a body. The usual complaints about the food were a chronic annoyance, and difficulties about employees were constant. These were dark days; days when I longed for dynamite or an earthquake as the shortest way out of all my troubles! I had to go on, however, and a good hunt would make me forget all my troubles for a time (Trudeau, 1915, p. 194).

The first caretakers were the Nortons, who retired in 1888. Trudeau hired Mrs. Julia A. Miller, who had run a very successful boarding house for tuberculosis patients in Saranac Lake. With her in charge, assisted by Frank Ingersoll, the sanitarium was run less like an extended family. It began to take on the organization and routinization required of a larger institution. This left Trudeau free to tend to his practice "and get some of my patients and friends to give us cottages from time to time" (Trudeau, 1915, p. 196).

That he had more freedom is revealed by Trudeau's notes in the case records which were written on a monthly schedule. Dr. Henry Sewall, in ill health himself, was recruited by Trudeau in return for board and lodging to live at the sanitarium (Trudeau, 1903, p. 126) in what Sewall called "the life saving winter of 1889" (letter with contribution from Denver, January 4, 1909). Presumably he lived on the campus and must have done considerable medical work. He signed many histories and physicals. At this point in time the records became considerably more systematic and comprehensive, reflecting the training of a younger physician.

Trudeau's treatment goal was to assist the body in fighting the disease. With rest and good food he built up the patient's resistance. Trudeau's cure depended on changing the person's way of living to prevent overexertion and relapse. For the remaining years of life the patient, who often looked very healthy, would have to be very careful not to overdo; otherwise, the disease would overcome the body's resistance.

By 1886 the sanitarium was on its feet and in business. There was little regimentation beyond that naturally occurring around the three meals that all ambulatory patients took together. Trudeau did not restrict patients a great deal beyond encouraging them to live out of doors as much as possible. As he visited the sanitarium at least monthly, he could not supervise their activities very closely.

In 1894 the sanitarium had nine new cottages, an open-air pavilion for recreation, an infirmary cottage, a library wing, and a home for the resident physician. In 1895 municipal water and electricity were installed. The hot water heating system was completed in 1898. Prior to this time medical residents had been single and used a room and office in the main building. In 1893 a new cottage allowed a married physician to work at the sanitarium. Dr. Irwin H. Hance and his wife were the first occupants, receiving three hundred dollars a year, plus the home and probably food supplies (Trudeau, 1915, p. 240). As far as patient care is concerned, a resident physician meant constant medical supervision.

One of the first changes that Trudeau made, once he had a waiting list, was to be selective about admissions. Those who had the best chance to recover were patients who had just contracted the disease. With the help of Dr. Baldwin's statistics, included in the annual reports of the Adirondack Cottage Sanitarium, Trudeau realized the best way to demonstrate convincing results was to treat more of the incipient cases. Therefore, he began a campaign to encourage doctors to recognize tuberculosis in its earliest stages so that treatment could begin immediately (Trudeau, 1901c).

Although Trudeau was willing to grant importance to the signs revealed by the stethoscope, he warned that, as these may appear too late, physicians should rely on the symptoms available to them from a thorough history.

Too much stress is laid upon the negative results of the microscopic examination and much valuable time lost on this account. Repeatedly, I see cases, beginning with hemoptysis and some failure of health—even when slight afternoon temperature is present, with or without some physical signs in the chest—where the patient is assured that he has not tuberculosis because one or two examinations of the expectoration have failed to reveal the presence of the bacillus (Trudeau, 1901c).

Trudeau had changed his mind about the microscope. When he first learned to stain and identify the bacillus in 1883, he was convinced that this technique provided ideal evidence for the disease. But it occurred too late to catch tuberculosis at the incipient stage, and he knew that was necessary to improve the likelihood of arresting the disease. While Trudeau respected the signs revealed by the new medical technology, he was aware of the limitations of these instruments and willing to rely on the symptoms he observed at earlier stages. From his experiments in the 1890s on animals and consenting patients Trudeau discovered another method for identifying tuberculosis at its early stage, the tuberculin test (Trudeau, 1901c).

He began to restrict admissions to the sanitarium to incipient cases. Obviously this brought some criticism from doctors who sent him patients who were refused admission. By this time he had a network of physicians who referred patients from all over the Northeast:

New York: Dr. James Alexander Miller, Dr. Linsley R. Williams, Dr. Henry James, Dr. Frederich J. Barrett [Dr. Loomis died in 1895.]

Boston: Dr. Francis H. Williams, Dr. Cleveland Floyd

Philadelphia: Dr. J. C. Wilson

Baltimore: Dr. H. M. Thomas, Dr. Louis Hamman (Trudeau, 1915, pp. 245–46).

All of these physicians examined people for the sanitarium without payment. Patients were sent to Saranac Lake to be seen by Dr. Trudeau for the sanitarium as well as for his private practice. If their cases were too advanced they would be sent to one of the cure cottages in the village.

In the late 1880s the village of Saranac Lake began a campaign to popularize the town as a health resort. The story of Trudeau's cure was published in newspapers as "The Miracle of the Wilderness." This legend and others by Murray, Stickler, et al. did a great deal to inform the general population of the rest cure in the Adirondacks (Caldwell, 1988, p. 43).

Beyond the confines of Little Red and its companion cottages on Mt. Pisgah, the steadily increasing numbers of health seekers coming to Saranac Lake were finding quarters in every type of structure from tents to the finest hotels. To keep pace with the need for space for these people (and, it must be acknowledged, to capitalize on that need), the entrepreneurs and healers of Saranac Lake (often in the guise of the same person—a nurse) began to open up houses as private, or non-institutional sanatoria. All but a few of these commercial private sanatoria had capacities of under twenty patients—most of them around a dozen or less—and the term "private sanitarium," or "private san," became virtually synonymous with the term "cure cottage." In a startlingly short time, the movement that had begun with Little Red began to transform the entire village into a cottage sanatorium. It would not be long before the village fathers would begin to publish promotional literature advertising Saranac Lake as the "Pioneer Health Resort" for the treatment of tuberculosis, which in fact it was (Gallos, 1985, p. 6).

As the Adirondack guides had once catered to wealthy "sports" wanting an experience in the great wilderness, their relatives created a health resort proud of its clean air and beautiful environment. "Sanitary Saranac" became a motto, implying that no one would ever spit on the street. When other physicians were reluctant to send patients to sanitoria because they now accepted the idea that tuberculosis was contagious, Trudeau's resident in 1891, Irwin Hance (1897), published his research on dust in the sanitarium's cottages.

Dr. Hance's research, which proved that the dust taken from all buildings at the institution, except in one instance, failed to infect guinea-pigs, and the published fact that ever since the Sanitarium was opened none of our employees or servants has been known to develop consumption, soon proved that the measures adopted to guard against infection there were efficacious for the protection of all residing at the institution (Trudeau, 1903c, p. 773).

Research was used to reassure patients and physicians and certify that sanitarium care was indeed sanitary. "Rest Hour" was sacred in the town, and during it even the radio station did not broadcast (Gallos, 1985, p. 168). When the railroad finally reached Saranac Lake, the town built a reception center to welcome these health seekers. Trudeau held office hours two days a week in Saranac Lake, while maintaining an active practice among the summer people at Paul Smith's, Hotel Saranac, St. Regis Lake, and other resorts of the wealthy. People who could afford resorts or private guides were advised to engage those accommodations. Others who were not in great need or were very sick were sent to cure cottages. Those who were in the incipient stage of tuberculosis and in financial need were accepted for the sanitarium, though they often had to wait to get in. Trudeau continued to advise those patients regardless of whether they were admitted to the sanitarium, and those who could afford it were charged a fee for board and room.

Their treatments varied as Trudeau and his colleagues learned or as various fads were publicized in the popular press and demanded by patients. But, always the foundation of the cure continued to be rest, fresh air, and nutritious food.

In the 1880s the routine of sanitarium care was very flexible, much was left up to the patients' judgment, and Trudeau functioned as a health educator. He taught patients the necessity of resignation—giving in to their chronic condition and learning to live with it. "The conquest of Fate comes not by rebellious struggle, but by acquiescence," he often said. Visiting them much as he saw his private patients who lived in family-owned camps or cure cottages, he taught them to live an outdoor life resting in the wilderness, to take care of their bodies, and to be sensitive to how they felt. If a walk in the woods resulted in fever, then they should rest and next time be less ambitious until they learned their limits. By gradual accommodation patients had to adapt to what their bodies could tolerate.

To those who did not recover, he was a sensitive and caring physician. Part of this sensitivity to people in general and patients in particular must have come from his personal experiences. His brother died in 1865, and his only daughter, Chatte, died in 1893 despite her father's efforts. Trudeau suffered a serious "abcess of the kidney" in the following winter of 1893–94 and occasional setbacks from tuberculosis all his life. When Ned died from pneumonia in 1904, another of Trudeau's episodes began and lasted until about 1906. Trudeau's life experiences did not seem to harden him but rather to sensitize him to the suffering of those for whom he cared. Some indication of the esteem that this caring engendered in the hearts of his friends and acquaintances is the support shown by the community when the Trudeaus buried Chatte and then Ned. The affection these townspeople, friends, and patients returned had first been given by this caring doctor and his wife.

As the sanitarium grew and as younger, differently trained physicians took over the day-to-day work, a routine and regimen developed.

The essential factors of the sanatorium method of treating tuberculosis I had labored to demonstrate . . . were all generally accepted and permanently established when Dr.

Brown became Resident Physician [1901], but the methods were crude, the discipline imperfect, and the records incomplete. He at once began to develop and perfect the medical department and its methods, and to bring them gradually to the high standard which they have attained during the past ten years. The simple and efficient rules of discipline, and thorough instruction of physicians, nurses, and patients, the accurate medical reports and the exhaustive post-discharge records of all patients since the institution started, the Medical Building with its facilities for the careful study of all cases on admission, and another scientific laboratory, all sprang into life as a result of Dr. Brown's insistent efforts for efficiency and continued progress. In addition, he found time to establish and edit for nine years *The Journal of the Outdoor Life*, which has rendered such far reaching service in the crusade against tuberculosis. As I had been only too glad to turn over the laboratory in Saranac Lake to Dr. Baldwin, it was an immense relief to me to place the medical department of the Sanitarium entirely in Dr. Brown's hands, since soon after his arrival my health and my capacity for work began steadily to fail (Trudeau, 1915, pp. 286–87).

The permissive and paternal teaching of the caring Dr. Trudeau was transformed into a more rigorous struggle with the disease, led by the physician. Lawrason Brown's principles were formalized in a medical textbook article in 1913:

The success of a physician in treating pulmonary tuberculosis depends largely on his ability to deal skillfully and individually with the physical, psychological, and sociological problems that arise with each patient. His former habits, pursuits, and idiosyncrasies must be carefully noted. He should be told at once that he has pulmonary tuberculosis, for the shock is soon over. The details of the treatment must be gone into fully and the importance of implicit obedience impressed. He should be told that in conscientious observance of minutiae lies health, and the reason for every rule should be made clear (Brown, 1913, p. 478).

It is likely that this rigorous and regimented approach developed gradually by trial and error. What is very clear is that the role of the doctor has changed from friendly educator to controlling leader (one wants to say, military commander). Brown described an appropriate daily schedule.

The details of the daily life for a patient may be stated simply as follows: 7:00, awake; milk (hot if desired) if necessary; cold sponge; 8:00, breakfast; 8:30, out-of-doors and at rest; 10:30, lunch when ordered; 11:00, exercise when needed; 1:00, dinner; indoors, not over one hour, less if possible; 2:00 to 4:00, absolute rest—no talking; sleep if possible; 3:30, lunch when ordered; 4:00 exercise when ordered; 6:00 supper; 7:00, outside on good nights; 9:00, lunch and bed. Once or twice a week a hot bath followed by a cold sponge (Brown, 1913, p. 478).

In this system the doctor regulated the patient through "orders" and exerted complete control over all aspects of a patient's life for a long period of time. Brown said, "Little can be expected from a 'cure' of less than three months, and the best results are those obtained after three or four years" (Brown, 1913, p. 464). He spelled out these ideas more explicitly in his book *Rules for Recovery from Pulmonary Tuberculosis: a Layman's Handbook*, published by Trudeau's old friend, Lea and Febiger of Philadelphia. The first edition was printed for patients in the sanitarium and in the village cure cottages. It eventually went through five more editions in 1916, 1919, 1923, 1928, and 1934. While the first two editions had a paternalistic tone, by the third edition Brown began to adopt Trudeau's style of treating the patient as an equal. He wrote in the introduction,

The day has come when the physician should look upon the patient, not as an ignorant child, but as a human being endowed with more or less mature intelligence; as one, in fact, who has a right to demand an explanation of the way certain effects follow certain causes. The physician of today must teach as well as serve; or better he must teach in order to serve most intelligently (Brown, 1919, pp. iii–iv).

So, after the turn of the century an outdoor life of rest in the healing woods was institutionalized into a rigorous process controlled by the physician. The original "cure" which the Adirondack guides had provided for Edward Trudeau in 1873 had become a medical campaign.

The key element in this care was control by the doctor, forcing patients to adjust to a new style of life and new conception of time. "Staff members emphasize the great length of time of the treatment and refuse to be pinned down to a precise estimate of just how long it will take" (Roth, 1963, p. xv). "The physician usually tells new patients to plan on at least a year in the hospital" (Roth, 1963, p. 7).

How patients felt in this new system can be illustrated from the diary of a former patient at another sanatorium.

At the Pines discipline was the most important factor (p. 45). . . . every thing that is not rest is exercise (p. 123). . . . As the rest in bed made almost everyone gain weight and stop coughing, only by laboratory test and x-rays could the Medical Director determine each patient's progress (p. 142). . . .
Of this progress we were told nothing. The only way we could tell whether we were getting well or dying was by the privileges we were granted. If we were progressing satisfactorily at the end of one month we were given the bathroom privilege and fifteen minutes a day reading-and-writing time. At the end of two months, if we continued to progress our reading-and writing time was increased to half an hour, we were allowed to read books and given ten minutes a day occupational therapy time. At the end of three months we were given a chest examination, along with other tests and if all was still well, we were given three hours time up, one hour occupational therapy time and could go to the movies (if chosen by the Charge Nurse) (MacDonald, 1948, p. 142).

Because two ingredients of the cure were still rest and fresh air, patients' beds had wheels so they could be pushed out on porches to breath the air at least eight hours each day, all year round. One former patient in the 1940s commented

"Many a night I slept out on the sleeping porches when it was 20, 30 below (zero) with an electric blanket and wearing a wool hat. You'd be boiling on the top from the electric blanket and on the bottom freezing where cold came through the bed" (Schultz, 1984, pp. 64–65). This led to a unique kind of architecture known as the "cure cottage," still visible in the village of Saranac Lake (Gallos, 1986).

Patients in some sanitoria were given a thermometer and required to plot their temperature daily, as fever was a sign of the disease. "A temperature of over 99 degrees F. in the case of males and over 99.6 degrees F in the case of females usually renders rest in bed imperative" (MacNalty, 1932, p. 80). Too much talking or reading during the day could cause an increase in fever if the patient was not careful. Constant normal temperature signified progress. The temperature chart and regular temperature readings focused attention upon a sign of the disease and gave the physician recorded evidence to back up clinical decisions. How the patient felt as a person was forgotten while these scientifically trained doctors focused upon data revealed by their technology. Medically supervised sanatorium care had come a long way since E. L. Trudeau drove his horse and buggy the fourteen miles from Paul Smith's every two weeks to ask his patients how they felt and to encourage them to take a walk in the woods if they felt they could handle it. The sanitarium had expanded its facilities, adding a library, workshop, bacteriology lab, X-ray facility, nursing school, and, the year after Trudeau's death, a summer institute for physicians. Because of the stigma attached to tuberculosis patients, many of the staff were recovered patients, as were the nursing students. Key staff members were provided housing to compensate for their low wages.

In Trudeau's lifetime the understanding of tuberculosis had changed a great deal. Lawrason Brown's book (1919) revealed the state of knowledge about 1915. The cause of tuberculosis was known, the tubercle bacillus. Dr. Brown taught patients that the bacillus "cannot live in sunshine and it cannot live in fresh air. . . . Thus, in a well lighted and ventilated room the tubercle bacillus is very speedily killed. This leads me to say that tuberculosis is a house disease. This means that it is practically never contracted out of doors but always in the house" (pp. 8–9). The source of the bacillus was human sputum and coughed particles from infected people. For this reason Brown advocated sweeping rooms, with "moist tea leaves or moist sawdust" to control dust, which was the chief carrier of the germs. Infected people were to use burnable tissues to catch the spray from coughing or burnable sputum boxes and wash their hands carefully. These preventive measures were especially necessary when a tuberculous family member lived in the same house.

While the primary source of the bacillus was dust in homes, another source, especially for children, was the milk from tuberculous cows. Therefore Brown argued that children should not drink milk from cows that failed the tuberculin test and that milk should be pasteurized. Also, he supported "good housing laws," encouraging healthy living conditions, open-air schools, and good air and good food to raise the resistance of children to all diseases. He argued that people should support their local boards of health, "for whatever improves the general health of the public reduces the amount of tuberculosis. For the same reason, better housing, better working conditions, better conditions in schools, open-air schools for children threatened with decline were important" (p. 170).

Climate had been thought to create tuberculosis free zones. The new belief in germs and understanding of contagion had changed these ideas. Brown reflected these changes:

Today, however, it is recognized that it is not climate but sparseness of population and difficulty of frequent communication with the outlying world that produces such zones, while density of population with the accompanying overcrowding under unsanitary and poor economic conditions plays a far more important part in reducing the individual resistance to the disease than any possible climatic condition (p. 136).

Such free zones were thought to provide valuable climates for treating tuberculosis. But that myth had been dispelled by new ideas,

The value of climate in the treatment of pulmonary tuberculosis rests today largely upon personal belief and experience, for much has been stated and little proved. Such widely divergent climates as the desert, the mountaintop or the mid-ocean are all good climates, and certain patients thrive wonderfully well under their influence. But it is now clearly recognized that proper treatment is more important than climate and, further, that there is no specific climate (pp. 136–37).

Brown dismissed the idea that tuberculosis was hereditary though he felt that "a predisposition to the disease may be inherited" from tuberculous parents. They should therefore observe strict precautions to prevent the bacillus from entering their children by the respiratory or alimentary routes.

He estimated that 75 percent of the people in New York City would react to a tuberculin test and therefore had "non-clinical or undeveloped tuberculosis." To prevent this from progressing to clinical tuberculosis he advised people to take care of themselves, "avoiding overwork, worry and disease."

Brown believed the cure could not be completed in a few months but required three or four years. To impress people with this, he noted that "thirty-eight percent of all patients who have been treated at the Trudeau Sanitarium have died." Food was essential, but only in amounts necessary to

hold his weight and strength. . . . The only way we can attack tuberculosis is by raising the body's powers of resistance to the highest point and then letting it fight against the disease. . . . We cannot cure a patient in six months, but we can get him in such shape that when he returns home he will know how to take the proper care of himself and to keep his body in such shape that it cannot only hold its own against the tubercle germ, but also fight against it and in three or four years overcome it (Brown, 1919, pp. 10–19).

The three great medicines, according to Brown, were "rest, food, and fresh air." Rest allowed the body to encapsulate the bacilli in the lungs, to "wall off the disease and so arrest it." "A patient is never injured by a six week rest in bed." The amount of rest was of course to be prescribed by the physician and judged according to the symptoms and condition of the patient (Brown, 1919, pp. 20–32).

Enough food was to be taken in a balanced diet to enable the patient to regain all lost weight. Milk, eggs, and cod-liver oil were prominent in regaining normal weight. Alcohol was "not necessary as a stimulant and rarely as a drug" (Brown, 1919, p. 52). "The kitchen is the only pharmacy that many patients should know" (Brown, 1913, p. 383). Smoking should be stopped or curtailed. Patients were encouraged to develop an "outdoor conscience," and cold air was considered more beneficial than warm (Brown, 1919, p. 69).

Patients were asked to rest in their beds on porches for at least eight to ten hours a day year round and to sleep in well-ventilated rooms. Those who had to continue working indoors were told to sleep out of doors all night (p. 12).

Throughout Brown's book for laymen (1919) many statements emphasized the role of the physician.

- The time that should be devoted to rest and the degree of rest varies, of course, with each individual and must be prescribed by his physician (p. 27).

- How long a patient should remain in bed depends entirely upon his condition and symptoms, points which only his physician can decide (p. 29).

- Nor must it be forgotten that the diet must be well balanced, and only the patient's physician can do this skillfully (p. 41).

- The question of when to get up must be decided by the physician (p. 94).

- The daily trip to the toilet is the first out-of-bed exercise permitted. It should be made every other day at first, but the physician's explicit permission must be obtained before this is begun. When this is well borne—all must depend upon the doctor's advice—sitting up in a reclining chair for one hour every other day may be begun (p. 95).

- As long as his muscles harden and his weight remains equal to or above his normal, exercise should be taken. Here, too, the advice of the physician is very necessary (p. 110).

- A tight cough at night is often helped by a cold pack on the chest and neck. However, before attempting this, one should get full details from his physician, how to apply it and whether or not it should be used in his case (p. 121).

- In any event a patient should never take any remedy without notifying his physician (p. 122).

Any layperson who read this book would become convinced that he or she would have to become completely dependent upon the physician.

What had changed since 1884, when Trudeau started the sanitarium? The germ theory of disease had slowly influenced medical thinking. By 1915, physicians were convinced that the tubercle bacillus existed and that people with tuberculosis were contagious. Their first line of defense against the white plague was prevention. All the preventive suggestions made by Hermann Biggs were followed by Trudeau and promoted by the National Association for the Study and Prevention of Tuberculosis and public health-minded physicians. The tuberculosis mortality rate had declined impressively in the last thirty years (see Figure 2.1). Prevention had a profound effect on decreasing mortality rates long before a specific cure was discovered. Physicians knew that one of the most effective ways to fight tuberculosis and many other diseases was to improve living and working conditions of all people.

Trudeau's belief in the sanitorium treatment, especially for incipient cases, gave hope to individuals who contracted the disease. The drastic change in their life style required by sanitorium care led to apparent cures for many. Devotion to an open-air lifestyle became a way-of-life for generations of people who had experienced healing in the woods. The sanitorium general treatment, of rest, open air, and good food, was tried in several forms. Trudeau's friend Vincent Bowditch used this treatment at a sanitorium for young women at Sharon, Massachusetts, in 1891 and demonstrated that climate was not an important factor. This convinced Massachusetts to open a state-supported sanitorium in 1898.

Another variation on sanitorium treatment was the tuberculosis class started by Joseph Pratt, a socially conscious physician, who had trained at Hopkins with Osler and practiced in Boston.

Pratt obtained financial aid from the Emmanuel Church and began his class in 1905; he combined the standard rest, diet, and fresh air treatment with close supervision of patients in the home and weekly meetings with a small "class" of patients. . . . He had each patient keep a notebook showing his daily temperature, diet, and hours in the open air. A spirit of friendly competition was encouraged. . . . Pratt believed that the success of the tuberculosis class was due to his insistence on absolute rest, plenty of fresh air, and diet, rather than the notebooks and weekly classes themselves (Teller, 1988, p. 80).

The idea caught on for a while, but by 1916 had dwindled to a few classes. Physicians like Pratt, "with great zeal, confidence, and patience" and interested in working with groups of patients, were not available.

Another form of sanitorium treatment was the day camp. In 1905,

The Boston Association for the Relief and Control of Tuberculosis opened a camp on Parker Hill. Patients came at 9:00 A.M. and spent the day in the open air, resting, reading, playing cards and knitting. A substantial dinner was served at noon and "luncheons" in the morning and afternoon. A physician and two nurses looked after the health of the 128 patients who attended (Teller, 1988, p. 81).

By 1911 there were "about thirty-seven" day camps in the Northeast. "Pittsburgh had a night camp where patients could have their pulse and temperature taken, get supper, sleep out of doors, and eat breakfast before returning to work" (Teller, 1988, p. 81). These camps attracted patients who would not otherwise have received care, but they were no substitute for full-time sanitorium treatment, which isolated infectious cases from their families and fellow workers.

One interesting but expensive experiment was the Home Hospital. In 1912, the New York Association for the improvement of the poor

selected seventeen families who agreed to follow the strict rules laid down to prevent infection, to occupy apartments in the East River Homes, a philanthropic model tenement. The building featured open exterior stairwells, a roof equipped with rest areas, shrubbery and a playground, and triple-hung windows extending from floor to ceiling. The Association provided relief, food, and even a housekeeper to do the heavy work in apartments where the mother was incapacitated. There was an outdoor school on the roof and close medical supervision by visiting physicians and a resident nurse. Unfortunately, the cost was high, and the Homestead Hospital was not initiated (Teller, 1988, p. 82).

Another form of sanitorium care was the "preventorium." Children from the homes of consumptives were accepted for three to six months.

The youngsters enjoyed life in the open air and abundant meals; they were taught cleanliness and hygiene as well as regular school subjects. During a child's stay at the preventorium, efforts were made to send the tuberculous family member to a sanatorium and improve the sanitary and hygiene conditions of the home. By 1916 there were eight preventoria in the United States with room for about 300 children, only a tiny fraction of those exposed (Teller, 1988, p. 110).

The idea of fresh air was applied to schools, with over 1,000 existing by 1916 (Teller, 1988, p. 114). These "open-air schools" offered food, fresh air, and rest to children who were malnourished and at risk for tuberculosis. Some of these applications of sanitorium methods were more successful than others, but cumulatively they must have had some effect, directly on the people involved and indirectly for publicity and education.

But the sanitorium still remained the best chance for recovery, especially for those who were identified at the earliest stages. And the responsibility of individuals for a healthy lifestyle and good health habits is experiencing new popularity today. Physicians are returning to holistic ideas that stress comprehending the totality of one's life and living experience in order to understand and treat disease.

13

The "Disappearance" of Tuberculosis

At Trudeau's death, the incidence rate for tuberculosis was still declining. It had dropped from 194.4 per 100,000 in 1900 to 140.1 by 1915. Prevention campaigns and public health laws in most cities and states required that consumptives be reported and isolated when this was possible. As many doctors refused to comply, eventually some states bribed them by paying for each reported case. Laws were passed against spitting in public places but were impossible to enforce. Posters prohibiting spitting did have an educational function. Dwellings of patients were disinfected, and people were taught to clean their rooms and remove dust. In its preventive crusade against the disease, the National Association for the Study and Prevention of Tuberculosis with its professional and lay members raised and spent $22,800,000 by 1915. There were 1,324 voluntary tuberculosis association affiliates in 1916 (Teller, 1988, p. 33). Its Christmas Seal campaign "provided tuberculosis associations with the money to expand their activities: to launch educational campaigns, open dispensaries, support tuberculosis nurses, promote open-air schools, and operate camps and sanitoria" (Teller, 1988, p. 34). The pasteurization of milk supplies became an accepted practice as did the testing of cows. Tuberculosis nurses went into homes to teach consumptives how to avoid spreading the germs to other members of their families and encouraged them to go to a sanitorium and protect their loved ones. In 1908, a British health officer, Dr. Arthur Newsholme, had lectured Congress, arguing that "isolation . . . was the most important element in the fall of the death rate from phthisis in England and Scotland" (Teller, 1988, p. 90). As the number of sanitoria for incipient cases and municipal hospitals that admitted advanced cases grew, more and more patients could be isolated.

Sanitoria had increased to 223 by 1916 with approximately 19,000 beds (p. 82) and 260 general hospitals provided another 16,000 beds. Trudeau's statistics had demonstrated that the sanitorium could give hope to incipient cases, but not for those who were far advanced.

Surgeons attempted to contribute to the campaign by recommending artificial pneumothorax and thoracoplasty. Both rested the lung by artificially collapsing it. While the procedures were widely used, evidence of their effectiveness was more testimonial than statistical.

Active screening for cases became a strategy with the examination of all school children, physical exams in the workplace, and the establishing of dispensaries and clinics. The Michigan Tuberculosis Survey "featured a traveling clinic which visited each county for a week; it was preceded by nurses who visited the local physicians to secure their cooperation and referrals, and by a publicity agent who involved the press and community leaders in the drive. Thousands took advantage of the clinics, and 2,914 cases of tuberculosis were uncovered; over half of these were classified as incipient" (Teller, 1988, p. 88). All of these preventive efforts were correlated in time with the declining tuberculosis death rate, but whether or not they were responsible for the decline from 140.1 in 1915 to 39.9 in 1945 has never been conclusively decided. "A decline in the mortality of an infectious disease can be due to four causes: (1) a decrease in the virulence of the infecting organism; (2) increased inherited resistance of the host caused by natural selection; (3) increased resistance because of improvement in the hygiene, nutrition, and environment of the host; and (4) specific measures to kill the infectious agent or prevent its spread" (Teller, 1988, p. 135).

By disinfecting rooms, controlling dust, preventing spitting in public places, encouraging that sputum of consumptives be burned, and isolating the contagious, the National Association did try to kill the bacillus and prevent its spread. By trying to improve hygiene, nutrition, and the environment of those most susceptible, preventive programs increased the resistance of individuals. But they were never able to make fundamental reforms in the society to prevent these conditions from developing again. With so many dying and so many displaying evidence of resistance to tuberculosis, natural selection of some kind may have occurred, but there is no evidence that the virulence of the bacilli changed. Nevertheless, the tuberculosis rate had declined impressively by 1945.

Streptomycin was first used in human experiments in 1946. Patients withlarge and growing lung lesions had promptly improved and occasionally healed. The drug operated almost passively interfering with the growth and reproduction of the tubercle bacillus rather than attacking it outright; it was largely ineffective during the considerable periods when the organism was dormant, and this meant that for effective treatment the dosage had to be continued for months. That in turn allowed resistant strains of bacteria to develop. At the Trudeau Sanatorium, an early study concluded that resistance began to appear during the fourth week of treatment and increased steadily thereafter (Caldwell, 1988, p. 265).

To counteract this resistance a new antibiotic, para-aminosalicylic acid (PAS) was combined with streptomycin by 1949. Another new drug, isonicotinic acid hydrazide (isoniazid) became the most effective drug after 1952. It inhibited the germs and killed them outright (Lowell, 1969, p. 25; Caldwell, 1988, p. 268). By 1967, the death rate from tuberculosis was down to 4.1 per 100,000, and over 500 tuberculosis sanitoria and countless cure cottages had either closed their doors or converted to other forms of institutional care including institutions for the aged, developmentally disabled, and prisons. The Trudeau Sanitorium had closed its doors in the fall of 1954, selling its property and using its endowment to establish the Trudeau Institute in Saranac Lake in 1964. This research facility is dedicated to pure biomedical research in chest and lung diseases and continues as one of the leading independent research institutes in the world.

THE REAPPEARANCE OF TUBERCULOSIS

Tuberculosis death rates remained so low that in 1989 federal health officials set the year 2010 as the target for eliminating tuberculosis in the United States. Almost as if to mock these human members of the biosphere, tuberculosis has reappeared.

In 1989, a man working in a Bath, Maine, shipyard developed cold symptoms and a cough. His doctor failed to test for tubercle bacilli and did not recognize that he had tuberculosis. For eight months he coughed while working the dusty interiors of ships and while socializing with his friends at a local tavern. Of 8,065 fellow workers, 417 were infected with the bacillus. Three of thirty tavern regulars were infected. "Among the 32 people with whom he both worked and socialized, 25, or 81 percent, were infected" (*The New York Times*, October 18, 1992).

Since 1985 the number of cases has begun to increase dramatically. The mortality rate for tuberculosis in the United States had increased to 10.5 per 100,000 by 1992, and 26,673 new cases were reported in that year. It is estimated that ten to fifteen million people are infected with the tuberculosis bacillus but are not sick (Office of Technology Assessment, 1993). Urban centers like Newark, New York, San Francisco, Miami, and Houston all had rates at least four times the national average, while Atlanta was the worst at nearly eight times the national average. In the rest of the world, especially in developing countries, tuberculosis remains a leading killer.

In retrospect, it appears that the low U.S. rates in the 60's and 70's diverted health officials toward more significant killers like heart disease and cancer. Even though treatment for tuberculosis could be completely effective "many patients did not complete the full course of drug treatment because the workers who supervised such therapy were laid off. Incomplete therapy fosters the development of drug-resistant strains, and when such patients returned to the community they spread drug-resistant tuberculosis to others . . . drug resistant tuberculosis has spread in at least 17 states. . . . In some outbreaks of drug-resistant tuberculosis, death rates have exceeded 80 percent . . . even when patients with drug-resistant tuberculosis end up in the hands of the top experts . . . the cure rate is only 50 percent (Altman, 1992a).

Because antibiotic treatment makes patients feel better in a few weeks, people who are homeless and scramble daily for a place to sleep and eat do not complete the year long course of treatment. At Harlem Hospital, a recent study showed that only one in ten patients completed the full course of treatment (Chowder, 1992). Though tuberculosis is one of the opportunistic infections that attacks AIDS sufferers, it is not limited to these men, women, and children. Inadequate health precautions have led to epidemics of tuberculosis in homeless shelters, community kitchens, prisons, nursing homes, and hospitals—wherever lack of sanitation, crowding, poor ventilation, and dust allow the bacilli to survive and spread. Though rates are higher among those who suffered from the neglect of our cities and the poor economic opportunities available in the 1980s and early 1990s, tuberculosis, like AIDS, can affect all social classes, especially health workers (Navarro, 1992). "The diagnosis of tuberculosis was made too late to save the life of Eleanor Roosevelt . . . who died of tuberculosis in 1962" (Altman, 1992a).

In the euphoria of the discovery of effective antibiotics, the social nature of tuberculosis was forgotten (Wright and Treacher, 1982). The preventive lessons that Trudeau and the National Association had taught at the beginning of this century were ignored. The result is that today we are being warned that tuberculosis could again become a major threat (Altman, 1992b). Whether a new cadre of socially conscious physicians will join equally interested lay persons to implement new prevention programs will probably depend upon the political climate.

The question of why tuberculosis "disappeared" was never resolved. It appears now that George Rosen was correct when he stated that the "decline in tuberculosis morbidity and mortality could be seen as an expression of an evolving biosocial process involving biologic characteristics of the human host, and environmental factors in dynamic equilibrium" (Berkman and Breslow, 1983, p. 8). In the 1980s and 1990s the human host and the environment were neglected. The bacillus has reemerged as a major threat. Perhaps the words of Hermann Biggs are appropriate. "Public health is purchasable. Within natural limits a community can determine its own death rate" (Teller, 1988, p. 135). Part of the genius of Edward Trudeau was that he recognized that tuberculosis was a biosocial process. Though he was enthusiastic about the possibilities of science and even eager to discover a cure, he recognized that prevention, early detection, and long-term treatment were what was needed.

THE ROLE OF MEDICAL SCIENCE

The cure for tuberculosis may exist, but we have seen that eradication of the disease is a complex biosocial process. Medical science is merely one of the players in this process, as the work of Edward Trudeau illustrates. The emerging science of bacteriology provided valuable concepts that Trudeau could use to develop belief in a method of cure that had allowed him to regain his health. His experience was that by following the wisdom of the Adirondack guides and resting in the woods, his tuberculosis was arrested. After several tragic periods in his life, Trudeau's health was restored by more rest in the woods. To explain what had happened, Edward Trudeau used medical science. The concept of "contagion" allowed Trudeau to understand how he must have caught the disease from his brother and later provided the justification for extensive programs of prevention and isolation. The concept of "germs" helped Trudeau identify the disease with great accuracy. With this laboratory skill he was able to convince his fellow physicians that germs did exist and connect his diagnostic acumen to the newly developing science of bacteriology. At a time when the elite in the medical profession nearly all had the experience of a year or two in Europe, Trudeau's familiarity with European research added to his stature. Being one of the first to culture the bacillus in his own laboratory, he developed the reputation of a basic scientist. At a time when Pasteur, Lister, Koch, and others were developing cures against other infectious diseases, the label "scientist" added greatly to his prestige among physicians and gave authority to his statements as a clinician.

The research that he published served several purposes. On the basis of his family, his performance at Physicians and Surgeons, and the recommendations of his mentors, Trudeau was invited to join the two leading organizations in his field, The American Climatological Association and the Association of American Physicians. He regularly read papers at the annual meetings of these groups as well as at those of the New York Academy of Medicine, the New York Pathological Society, and others. Trudeau's famous rabbit experiment presented to the American Climatological Association, legitimated sanitorium treatment and its goal of increasing the body's ability to resist the bacilli.

Trudeau was a living testimony that the outdoor method "cured" tuberculosis. His "scientific research evidence," combined with the popular press and medical belief in the healing power of nature, gave further credibility to his outdoor method. Already popular with the wealthy, the Adirondack woods was opened up to those without funds by the Adirondack Cottage Sanitarium. Trudeau's colleagues willingly sent him patients. Those who could afford hotels or cure cottages were seen by Trudeau privately. Those incipient cases who could not, were admitted to the sanitarium.

Another function of Trudeau's experimental work was to give the impression that the sanitarium was the place where the very latest research findings were being tested. It was assumed that the accuracy and precision of the laboratory would carry over to the sanitarium. Though he was very careful to test remedies on animals, Trudeau did try some remedies on patients, such as hydrofluoric acid, sulphur, hot air, and creosote in the cabinet treatment. When tuberculin became available, Trudeau was one of the first to treat patients with the new remedy. That it did not work may not have been as important as the fact that his sanitarium used tuberculin, something for which publicity had created great demand. When Trudeau published the results of his tuberculin injections, he used the negative results to focus attention upon the positive results being achieved by the outdoor life cure at the sanitarium. In making this contrast he was able to divert much of the intense enthusiasm for tuberculin toward sanitorium care.

Trudeau's attempt to develop a vaccine and to search for a method to immunize animals kept his laboratory and the sanitarium at the forefront of tuberculosis studies. He was a knowledgeable authority very capable of convincing others of the value of the "facts" as he saw them. Although the results he presented were not spectacular, they were certainly better than complete failure. As he began to emphasize early identification of incipient cases and limit admissions to such cases, more impressive results could be demonstrated. Whether the open-air treatment really worked was not a question to be asked.

Trudeau's rabbit experiment was evidence that it did. Experiments on humans were out of the question. Whether those incipient cases that were "cured" and "arrested" would have experienced the same results if they had not been sent to a sanitorium was never tested. Bowditch's experiment in Massachusetts and other open-air attempts throughout the country suggested that a sanitorium setting might not be necessary. But rest, good food, and an open-air life in the woods had a romantic and popular appeal that is with us even today.

This may account for the scientific and medical acclaim that Trudeau received, but there were expressions of love given at several points in Trudeau's life, especially at the funerals of Chatte and Ned and at Trudeau's funeral. That acclaim came from Trudeau's character. Motivated by the desire "to sometimes cure, often help, and always console," Trudeau conveyed a sincere kind of caring to his patients. Those who improved were grateful for the result and expressed it in many ways. Those who did not improve felt that all that could be done by medical science and human effort had been done. Many of these patients and their families were grateful also. That Trudeau's sanitarium work was performed without direct remuneration was further evidence of his caring and concern for others. Trudeau championed the cause of prevention despite the protests of some medical people, and he was willing to work with non-medical scientists and lay persons in the crusade against tuberculosis. For these efforts as a socially conscious physician, he was recognized by everyone and honored by the tributes at his death.

Bibliography

Ackerknecht, E. H. 1967. "A Plea for a Behaviorist Approach in Writing the History of Medicine." *Bulletin of the History of Medicine* 22, pp. 211–14.

Altman, Lawrence K. 1992a. "Drug-Resistant TB Makes U.S. Rethink Elimination Program." *The New York Times,* February 11.

———. 1992b. "Top Scientist Warns Tuberculosis Could Become Major Threat." *The New York Times*, February 11.

Baldwin, Edward R. 1913. "Tuberculosis: History and Etiology." In William Osler and Thomas McCrae (eds.), *Modern Medicine in Theory and Practice,* pp. 287–338. Philadelphia: Lea and Febiger.

———. 1900. "Some Results of the Climatic and Sanitorium Treatment of Tuberculosis in the Adirondacks." *Transactions of the New York State Medical Society.* Unpublished. Saranac Lake: Trudeau Institute Library.

———. 1916. "Dr. Trudeau, the Investigator." *Johns Hopkins Hospital Bulletin* 27(302) (April), pp. 96–107.

Bates, Barbara. 1992. *Bargaining for Life*. Philadelphia: University of Pennsylvania Press.

Berkman, Lisa F., and Lester Breslow. 1983. *Health and Ways of Living*. New York: Oxford University Press.

Biggs, Hermann M. 1910. "Dr. Trudeau as a Pioneer in the Anti-Tuberculosis Movement." *Journal of the Outdoor Life* 7(6) (June), pp. 163–65.

Blades, Brooke S. 1978. "Doctor Williams' privy." In *New England Historical Archaeology*, pp. 56–63.

Brown, Lawrason. No date. "A Tuberculosis Chronology." Trudeau Institute, unpublished.

———. 1913. "The Symptoms, Diagnosis, Prognosis, Prophylaxis and Treatment of Tuberculosis" in William Osler and Thomas McCrae (eds.), *Modern Medicine in Theory and Practice,* pp. 376–521. Philadelphia: Lea and Febiger.

———. 1931. "Trudeau." *Journal of the Outdoor Life* 28 (May).

————. 1919. *Rules for the Recovery from Pulmonary Tuberculosis: A Layman's Handbook of Treatment,* 3d ed. Philadelphia: Lea and Febiger. [The first edition was published in 1915, the 6th edition in 1934].

Burke, R. M. 1938. *A Historical Chronology of Tuberculosis.* Springfield: Charles C. Thomas Publishers.

Cadbury, Warder H. 1989. "Introduction and Notes" to W. H. H. Murray. *Adventures in the Wilderness.* Adirondack Museum: Syracuse University Press.

Caldwell, Mark. 1988. *The Last Crusade.* New York: Atheneum.

Chalmers, Steven. 1915. "The Beloved Physician: An Appreciation of Edward Livingston Trudeau." Privately published.

————. 1916. *The Beloved Physician: Edward Livingston Trudeau.* Boston: Houghton-Mifflin Co.

Chowder, Ken. 1992. "How TB Survived Its Own Death to Confront Us Again." *Smithsonian.* November, pp. 180f.

Clapesattle, Helen. 1984. *Dr. Webb of Colorado Springs.* Boulder: Colorado Associated University Press.

Clark, Alonzo. 1853. "Annual Address to the New York State Medical Society and Members of the Legislature." February.

Coe, Rodney M. 1970. *Sociology of Medicine.* New York: McGraw-Hill.

Cooter, Roger. 1982. "Anticontagionism and History's Medical Record." In P. Wright and A. Treacher (eds.), *The Problem of Medical Knowledge,* pp. 87–108. Edinburgh: Edinburgh University Press.

Cousins, Norman. 1979. *The Anatomy of an Illness as Perceived by the Patient.* New York: W. W. Norton.

Dodge, Henry N. 1867–68. "Notes on Lectures," College of Physicians and Surgeons. Archives of Columbia College of Physicians and Surgeons.

Donaldson, Alfred L. 1915. "Edward L. Trudeau." *The New York Times Magazine.* November 21.

————. 1921. *A History of the Adirondacks,* vol. 1. Fleischmanns, New York: Purple Mountain Press. Unabridged reprint of the 1921 edition published by the Century Co.

Duquette, John J. 1977. "A Biographical Sketch of Alfred Lee Donaldson." In A. L. Donaldson. *A History of the Adirondacks,* vol. 1. Fleischmanns, New York: Purple Mountain Press. Unabridged reprint of the 1921 edition published by the Century Co.

Fleming, Donald. 1987. *William H. Welch and the Rise of Modern Medicine.* Baltimore: Johns Hopkins Press.

Flexner, Simon. 1910. "Edward L. Trudeau, Physician, Investigator, and Optimist." *Journal of the Outdoor Life* 7(6) (June), pp. 169–72.

Flint, Austin. 1867. *A Treatise on the Principles and Practice of Medicine.* Philadelphia: Henry C. Lea.

————. 1874. *Essays on Conservative Medicine and Kindred Topics.* Philadelphia: Henry C. Lea.

Gallos, P. 1986. *Cure Cottages of Saranac Lake.* Saranac Lake: Historic Saranac Lake.

Gould, George M. 1892. Letter to Edward L. Trudeau, Adirondack Room of Saranac Lake Public Library.

Halleck, Fitz Greene. 1910. "Early Hunting Days with Dr. Trudeau." *Journal of the Outdoor Life* 7(6) (June), pp. 177–78.

Hance, Irwin H. 1897. "A Further Study of Tuberculosis Infection of Dust." *Medical Record* 51(7) (February 13).

Handlin, Oscar. 1987. "Editor's Preface." In Donald Fleming, *William H. Welsh and the Rise of Modern Medicine.* Baltimore: Johns Hopkins Press.

Harrod, K. E. 1959. *Man of Courage: The Story of Dr. Edward L. Trudeau*. New York: Julian Messner.

Harvey, A. McGehee. 1986. *The Association of American Physicians 1886–1986*. Baltimore: Waverly Press.

Haskell, Helen Woolford. 1981. *The Middletown Privy House*. Columbia: University of South Carolina Institute of Archaeology and Anthropology, Popular Series 1.

Holden, Constance. 1992. "Random Samples." *Science* 257 (July 3), p. 26.

Hotaling, Mary B. 1991. "Edward Livingston Trudeau, M.D.: Pioneer Medical Scientist." Manuscript. Historic Saranac Lake.

House, H. D. 1934. *Wild Flowers*. New York: Macmillan.

Houser, R. No date. "Selected Highlights from the Chronology of Tuberculosis." Manuscript. New York State Health Department, Bureau of Tuberculosis Control.

Hutchison, James C. 1865–66. "Notes taken at the College of Physicians and Surgeons," Regular Course of Lectures. Archives of Columbia College of Physicians and Surgeons.

James, Walter B. 1916. "Trudeau, the Physician." *Johns Hopkins Hospital Bulletin* 27(302) (April), pp. 96–107.

Kaufman, M. 1971. *Homeopathy in America*. Baltimore: Johns Hopkins Press.

Kett, Joseph F. 1965. *The Formation of the American Medical Profession*. New Haven: Yale University Press.

Kevles, D. J., J. L. Sturchio, and P. T. Carroll. 1980. "The Sciences in America, Circa 1880." *Science* 209 (July 4), pp. 27–32.

King, L. S. 1982. *Medical Thinking*. Princeton: Princeton University Press.

Koch, Robert. 1891. "Koch's Treatment of Tuberculosis." *The American Journal of the Medical Sciences* 101(2) (February), pp. 171–79.

Krause, A. K. 1916. "Reflections on Dr. Trudeau." *Medical Pickwick*. Saranac Lake: Trudeau Institute Library.

Latour, Bruno. 1988. *The Pasteurization of France*. Translated by Alan Sheridan and John Law. Cambridge: Harvard University Press.

Loomis, A. L. 1895. "Obituary." *Harper's Weekly,* January, pp. 137–38.

Loomis, H. P. 1890. "A Study of the Koch Method in Berlin." *Medical Record* 38(26) (December 27), pp. 721–24.

Lowell, A. M. 1969. "Tuberculosis Morbidity and Mortality and Its Control." *Tuberculosis*. Part 1. Cambridge: Harvard University Press. Published by the American Public Health Association.

Lusk, Wm. B. 1915. "Edward L. Trudeau." *The Churchman,* December 18, pp. 37–38.

MacDonald, B. 1948. *The Plague and I*. Philadelphia: J. P. Lippincott Company.

MacNalty, A. S. 1932. "A Report on Tuberculosis. Including an Examination of the Results of Sanatorium Treatment." In *Reports on Public Health and Medical Subjects,* no. 64. London: His Majesty's Stationery Office.

Murray, W. H. H. 1869. *Adventures in the Wilderness*. Republished 1989 by the Adirondack Museum and Syracuse University Press.

Navarro, Mireya. 1992. "Study Finds TB Danger Even in Low-Risk Groups." *The New York Times,* October 18.

Nordhoff, Charles. 1875. *The Communistic Societies of the United States*. New York: Schocken Books. Reprinted in 1965.

Office of Technology Assessment. 1993. *The Continuing Challenge of Tuberculosis*. Washington, D.C.: U.S. Government Printing Office.

O'Hara, Leo J. 1989. *An Emerging Profession: Philadelphia Doctors, 1860–1890*. New York: Garland.

Osler, William. 1910. "Edward L. Trudeau—An Appreciation." *Journal of the Outdoor Life*
    7(6), (June) pp. 162–63.
Purdy, A. E. M. 1890. *Lectures on the Practice of Medicine by Alonzo Clark*. Given to the New
    York Academy of Medicine on February 24, 1890. Archives of the New York Medical
    Society.
Reiser, S. J. 1982. *Medicine and the Reign of Technology*. New York: Cambridge University
    Press.
Robinson, Beverley. 1889. "Creosote as a Remedy in Phthisis Pulmonalis." *American Journal
    of the Medical Sciences* 48(1) (January), pp. 1–15.
Rosen, G. (ed.). 1983. *The Structure of American Medical Practice 1875–1941*. Philadelphia:
    University of Pennsylvania Press.
Rosenberg, Charles E. 1962. *The Cholera Years*. Chicago: University of Chicago Press.
———. 1967. "The Practice of Medicine in New York a Century Ago." *Bulletin of the History
    of Medicine* 41, pp. 223–53.
———. 1961. *No Other Gods: On Science and American Social Thought*. Baltimore: Johns
    Hopkins University Press.
Roth, J. A. 1963. *Timetables*. Indianapolis: Bobbs-Merrill.
Ryan, Frank. 1992. *The Forgotten Plague*. Boston: Little, Brown.
Scrapbook 10. From a series of Scrapbooks containing clippings about the Adirondack Cottage
    Sanitarium. Saranac Lake, New York: Trudeau Institute Library.
Shultz, Rebecca. 1984. "The Trudeau Institute." *Adirondack Life* (January/February), pp.
    46f.
Smith, Paul. 1910. "Dr. Trudeau's First Winter in the Adirondacks." *Journal of the Outdoor Life*
    7(6) (June), pp. 175–76.
Spiegelman, M., and C. L. Erhardt. 1974. "Mortality in the United States by Cause." In C. L.
    Erhardt and J. E. Berlin (eds.), *Morbidity and Mortality in the United States*. Cambridge:
    Harvard University Press.
Starr, Paul. 1982. *The Social Transformation of American Medicine*. New York: Basic Books.
Stickler, Joseph W.(ed.) 1886. *The Adirondacks as a Health Resort*. New York: G. P. Putnam's
    Sons.
Tauber, Alfred L., and Leon Chernyak. 1991. *Metchnikoff and the Origins of Immunology*. New
    York: Oxford University Press.
Taylor, Robert. 1986. *Saranac: America's Magic Mountain*. Boston: Houghton-Mifflin.
Teller, Michael E. 1988. *The Tuberculosis Movement*. Westport, Conn.: Greenwood Press.
Thomas, Henry M. 1916. "Memorial to Edward L. Trudeau." *Proceedings of the Laennec
    Society*. Johns Hopkins Hospital. January 24.
———. 1885. "An Experimental Research upon the Infectiousness of Non-Bacillary Phthisis."
    American Journal of the Medical Sciences 90, pp. 361–65.
Trudeau, Edward L. 1886. "A Case Illustrating the Value of the Tubercle Bacillus as an Aid to
    an Early Diagnosis in Phthisis." *New York Medical Journal* 44, p. 464.
———. 1887a. "Environment in its Relation to the Progress of Bacterial Invasion in Tubercu-
    losis." *Transactions of the American Climatological Association* 4, pp. 131–36.
———. 1887b. "Sulphretted Hydrogen versus the Tubercle Bacillus." *Medical News* 51
    (November 12), p. 570.
———. 1888. "Hydrofluoric Acid as a Destructive Agent to the Tubercle Bacillus." *Medical
    News* 52 (May 5), pp. 486–90.
———. 1889. "Hot-Air Inhalations in Pulmonary Tuberculosis." *Medical News* 55 (September
    28), pp. 337–38.
———. 1890a. "The Contagiousness of Influenza." *Medical News* 56 (February 15), pp.
    185–86.

———. 1890b. "Some Cultures of the Tubercle Bacillus Illustrating Variations in Its Mode of Growth and Pathogenic Properties." *Transactions of the Association of American Physicians* 5, pp. 183–90.

———. 1890c. "An Experimental Study of Preventive Inoculation in Tuberculosis." *Medical Record* 38(21), November 22, pp. 565–68.

———. 1891. "Variations in the Mode of Growth of Tubercle Bacilli." *Proceedings of the New York Pathological Society* 22, pp. 75–77.

———. 1892a. "Results of the Employment of Tuberculin and Its Modifications at the Adirondack Cottage Sanitarium." *Medical News* 61, pp. 298–300.

———. 1892b. "The Treatment of Experimental Tuberculosis by Koch's Tuberculin, Hunter's Modification and Other Products of the Tubercle Bacillus." *Medical News* 61(10), (September 3), pp. 253–58.

———. 1892c. "Observations in Adirondack Cottage Hospital." *Transactions of the New York Academy of Medicine 8, pp. 163–67.*

———. 1893. "Eye Tuberculosis and Antitubercular Inoculation in the Rabbit." *Medical Record* 58, pp. 97–98.

———. 1894. "A Report of the Ultimate Results Obtained in Experimental Eye-Tuberculosis by Tuberculin Treatment and Anti-Tuberculosis Inoculation." *Medical News* 65 (September 29), pp. 346–48.

———. 1897a. "The Tuberculin Test in Incipient and Suspected Pulmonary Tuberculosis." *Medical News* 70(22) (May 29), pp. 687–90.

———. 1897b. "Remarks on Artificial Immunity in Tuberculosis." *British Medical Journal* 2, pp. 1849–50.

———. 1897c. "Sanitaria for the Treatment of Incipient Tuberculosis." *Medical Record* 65 (February 27), pp. 276–81.

———. 1897d. "Sanataria for the Treatment of Incipient Tuberculosis." *New York Medical Journal* 65 (February 27), pp. 276–81.

———. 1899a. "The Present Aspect of Some Vexed Questions Relating to Tuberculosis, with Suggestions for Future Research Work." *Bulletin of Johns Hopkins Hospital* 10 (July), pp. 121–26.

———. 1899b. "The Adirondack Cottage Sanitarium for the Treatment of Incipient Pulmonary Tuberculosis." *The Practitioner* 62, pp. 131–46.

———. 1900a. "The First People's Sanatorium in America for the Treatment of Pulmonary Tuberculosis." *Zeitschrift fur Tuberkulose Und Heilstattenwesen* 1, pp. 230–39.

———. 1900b. "The Sanitarium Treatment of Incipient Pulmonary Tuberculosis and Its Results." *Medical News* 76, pp. 852–57.

———. 1900c. "The Sanitarium Treatment of Incipient Pulmonary Tuberculosis and Its Results." *Transactions of the Association of American Physicians* 15, pp. 36–47.

———. 1901a. "The History and Work of the Saranac Laboratory for the Study of Tuberculosis." *Bulletin of the Johns Hopkins Hospital* 12(126), pp. 271–75. Price 15 cents.

———. 1901b. "The Importance of a Recognition of the Significance of Early Tuberculosis in Relation to Treatment." *Medical News* 78(26) (June 29), pp. 1013–14.

———. 1901c. "The Importance of a Recognition of the Significance of Early Tuberculosis in Relation to Treatment." *Transactions of the Association of American Physicians* 16, pp. 113–18.

———. 1903a. "Artificial Immunity in Experimental Tuberculosis." *Transactions of the Association of American Physicians* 18, pp. 97–107.

———. 1903b. "Artificial Immunity in Experimental Tuberculosis." *New York Medical Journal* and *Philadelphia Medical Journal* (consolidated) 78(3) (July), pp. 105–10.

————. 1903c. "The History of the Tuberculosis Work at Saranac Lake." *Medical News* 83(17), (October 24), pp. 769–80.

————. 1903–4. "The History of the Tuberculosis Work at Saranac Lake, New York." *Henry Phipps Institute, First Annual Report,* pp. 121–40.

————. 1905a. "Address of the President." *Medical News* 87(1), (July), pp. 1–3.

————. 1905b. "Address of the President." *National Association for the Study and Prevention of Tuberculosis. Transactions.* No. 1, pp. 13–19.

————. 1905c. "Address of the President." *Transactions of the Association of American Physicians,* 20, pp. 1–3.

————. 1909a. "Animal Experimentation and Tuberculosis." *Journal of the Outdoor Life* 6(3), (March), pp. 61–62.

————. 1909b. *Century Magazine.* August.

————. 1910a. "Some Personal Reminiscences of Robert Koch's Two Greatest Achievements in Tuberculosis." *Journal of the Outdoor Life* 7(July), pp. 189–92.

————. 1910b. "Address before the 8th Congress of American Physicians and Surgeons," May 2. Washington, D.C. Scrapbook 10, p. 54. Trudeau Institute.

————. 1915. *Autobiography.* Garden City, N.Y.: Doubleday.

Trudeau, Edward L., and Edward R. Baldwin. 1895. "A Chemical and Experimental Research on 'Antiphthisin (Kleb's).' " *Medical Record* 48 (December 21), pp. 871–74.

————. 1898a. "Experimental Studies on the Preparation and Effects of Antitoxins for Tuberculosis. Part I." *American Journal of the Medical Sciences* 116, pp. 692–707.

————. 1898b. "A Resumé of Experimental Studies on the Preparation and Effects of Antitoxic Serum in Tuberculosis." *Transactions of the Association of American Physicians* 13, pp. 111–23.

————. 1899. "Experimental Studies on the Preparation and Effects of Antitoxins for Tuberculosis. Part II." *American Journal of the Medical Sciences* 116, pp. 56–76.

Twaddle, A., and R. Hessler. 1987. A Sociology of Health, 2d ed. New York: Macmillan.

Waksman, Selman A. 1964. *The Conquest of Tuberculosis.* Berkeley: University of California Press.

Warner, John H. 1986. *The Therapeutic Perspective: Medical Practice, Knowledge, and Identity in America, 1820–1885.* Cambridge: Harvard University Press.

Weigert, Louis. 1888. "A New Method of Treating Consumption by Inhalation of Hot Dry Air." *Medical Record* 34(24) (December 15), pp. 693–95.

Wright, Peter, and Andrew Treacher (eds.). 1982. *The Problem of Medical Knowledge: Examining the Social Construction of Medicine.* Edinburgh: Edinburgh University Press.

Index

About the Author

David L. Ellison is Associate Professor of Medical Sociology at Rensselaer Polytechnic Institute. Among his earlier publications is *The Bio-Medical Fix* (Greenwood Press, 1978).

ISBN 0-313-29005-9

EAN

HARDCOVER BAR CODE